The Fibre Effect

The surprising (and easy) way to transform your health

EMMA BARDWELL

Vermilion
LONDON

VERMILION

UK | USA | Canada | Ireland | Australia
India | New Zealand | South Africa

Vermilion is part of the Penguin Random House group of companies
whose addresses can be found at global.penguinrandomhouse.com

Penguin Random House UK
One Embassy Gardens, 8 Viaduct Gardens, London SW11 7BW

penguin.co.uk

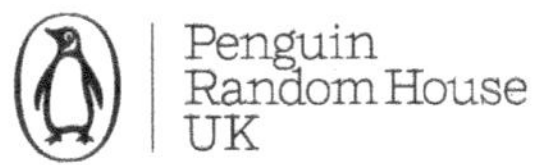

Penguin
Random House
UK

First published by Vermilion in 2026

1

Typeset by seagulls.net

Printed and bound in Great Britain by Clays Ltd, Elcograf S.p.A.

The authorised representative in the EEA is Penguin Random House Ireland,
Morrison Chambers, 32 Nassau Street, Dublin D02 YH68

A CIP catalogue record for this book is available from the British Library

ISBN 9781785046278

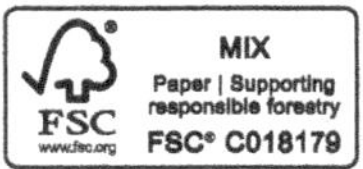

Penguin Random House is committed to a sustainable future
for our business, our readers and our planet. This book is
made from Forest Stewardship Council® certified paper.

Raf, thanks for the consistently loud (and proud)
feedback that fibre works

Disclaimer

The information provided in this book is for general guidance only and is not intended as medical advice or to replace the care of a qualified healthcare professional. Some of the dietary suggestions may not be appropriate for individuals with specific gastro-intestinal conditions or other health issues. Please consult an appropriately qualified health professional before making any changes to your diet, lifestyle or treatment plan to ensure that such changes are safe and suitable for your individual needs.

Contents

PART ONE:
UNLOCKING THE POWER OF FIBRE

PART TWO:
FIBRE ON YOUR PLATE

The Recipes

PART THREE:
YOUR FIBRE TOOLKIT

Introduction

Say hello to your new favourite f-word

The fact that you've picked out this book means you already have an inkling that fibre is important, but you might not necessarily think of it as a superstar. If you follow me on social media, you'll have heard me wax lyrical about fibre's role in gut health, mood, immunity, weight loss, blood sugar control and even how good your skin looks. I also discussed it as one of the three crucial pillars for health in my previous book, *The 30g Plan*. Yet, in the UK, 96% of us still aren't eating the recommended 30g a day. Sadly, despite its impressive CV, fibre rarely gets the spotlight it deserves – too often cast as a rather bland support act, never the star of the show.

I'm here to change that.

By the end of *The Fibre Effect*, you'll see fibre for what it truly is: the ultimate superfood. But not in a gimmicky way. Fibre isn't a fleeting fad you'll forget all about after a few weeks. It's a forever thing – something you'll focus on for the rest of your life, hopefully. Don't worry, it's not complicated, expensive or hard to find. Fibre is in real, everyday food. It's abundant, accessible, can taste next-level (honestly, I'll show you how!) and – best of all – it has the power to utterly transform your health.

Why fibre is the ultimate superfood

Let me quickly show you why fibre is so deserving of a superstar status.

1. Fibre does a *lot* more than 'keep you regular'.

Most people think of fibre as your gut's broom, helping to sweep food along your digestive tract. And while that's true, it's just a small part of what fibre does for us. Fibre feeds your gut microbes, balances your blood sugar, helps manage cholesterol, supports healthy weight and even reduces the risk of diseases like type 2 diabetes, heart disease and certain cancers. In fact, when scientists try to pin down a single dietary factor that explains why some people live longer, healthier lives, it's fibre that keeps showing up.

2. Fibre is everywhere (and it's affordable).

Unlike faddy wellness foods that are expensive and hard to find, fibre is found in the basics: fruit, vegetables, legumes (beans, chickpeas, lentils), wholegrains, nuts and seeds. You don't need a specialist shop or an expensive subscription to some elite supplement; you just need to eat more of these everyday foods that are available in any supermarket. If you're worried this sounds like one more thing to cram into your already time-poor life, you can rest easy. I'm going to show you how simple – not to mention diverse and wonderfully delicious – it can be. And for the omnivores among you, no, I'm not going to make you give up meat.

3. Fibre works with your body, not against it.

Dietary advice can sometimes feel like punishment: cutting things out, restricting, weighing and measuring. Fibre is different. The simple act of adding more fibre to your meals improves your health, naturally crowds out less-helpful foods, keeps you feeling full for longer and nudges you towards more balance without you even really noticing. It's less about *ex*clusion, more about *in*clusion.

4. Feel the fibre effect – now and for years to come.

The best part about fibre is you don't have to wait years to feel the benefits. More fibre at breakfast can mean steadier energy by lunchtime. After increasing your fibre intake for a week or two, you may well notice an improvement in digestion, a reduction in bloating and an overall feeling of being lighter. Stick with it for months and years and you're stacking the odds in favour of lifelong health. Trust me, few other ingredients can claim that kind of immediate *and* far-reaching impact.

In a nutshell, *The Fibre Effect* is about making fibre simple, practical and doable in your everyday life. No jargon. No complicated formulas. Just a clear understanding of what it is, why it matters and how to make it work for you. Because once you see how deeply fibre connects to everything – from digestion and mood to hormones and lifespan – you won't be able to get enough of this superstar ingredient. I strongly believe that fibre isn't just part of the wellbeing picture; it's the framework that holds it all together.

The fibre effect timeline: When you'll start feeling the benefits

If you're anything like me, you're always keen to see results when you make dietary changes. To give you a sense of the journey, here's a rough timeline of what happens when you up your fibre game:

- **Steadier energy [within hours]**
  That mid-morning crash after breakfast will be a thing of the past. Fibre helps blunt the elevation in blood sugar that can often follow less-balanced meal choices like granola or a slice of toast and jam. *The Fibre Effect* will show you how to kick off the day so you stay fuelled, focused and upbeat.

- **Feeling more full after meals and less 'hangry' [24 hours]**
  Fibre adds bulk and slows digestion, so food stays in your stomach for longer. You'll likely feel pleasantly satisfied straight after meals rather than constantly scanning the kitchen for your next fix. And, with more stable blood sugars, you can also expect to experience a generally calmer headspace, fewer cravings and a lovely quieting of 'food noise'

so you can think about life, rather than constantly obsessing over what you're going to eat.

- **Changes in gut bacteria [24–48 hours]**
  Eating more fibre means your gut microbes get fed, too. According to medical journal *Nature*, populations of fibre-loving species can increase within 24–48 hours, while less-helpful microbes fade into the background. Think of it as a re-wilding of your gut. An improved gut microbiome can support immunity, lower inflammation and even influence mood.

- **More regular digestion [within days]**
  If constipation or sluggishness is an onging issue, you'll probably notice gentler, easier bowel movements. Honestly, nothing beats 'poophoria' – the hugely life-affirming joy of having an effortless, satisfying poo!

- **Feeling lighter, more energetic and with less bloating (yes, really!) [within weeks]**
  Not from calorie-cutting, but because your body is running on steadier fuel and flooding your body with micronutrients from the increased consumption of fibre from plants. And yes, more complete, satisfying trips to the toilet will also leave you feeling noticeably lighter and more comfortable. Once your gut adapts to more fibre (I'll guide you through this starting on p. 100), many people notice less discomfort and less bloating than before, too.

- **Improved cholesterol, blood pressure and other health markers [4+ weeks]**
  Many of the people I work with see improvements in blood tests in just a few weeks, including lowering LDL, the 'bad' cholesterol. This will depend on whether you have any other health conditions affecting your cholesterol. If you suffer from high blood pressure, you may see this lower, too. Increased fibre means your blood vessels, liver and even your immune system are all quietly benefitting in the background, and markers of disease risk are improving.

- **Stronger gut lining and more efficient excretion of toxins [8 weeks]**
  One of the jobs your gut bacteria has is to help repair and protect the barrier in your intestines, making it stronger and more resilient against inflammation. Of course, we're all unique, so changes are highly individual, but one study showed changes in inflammatory markers after as little as eight weeks of eating more fibre. Your body also uses fibre to help expel things from your gut that it doesn't want hanging around: excess hormones, toxins and even potentially microplastics – helping you excrete them instead of letting them build up.

- **Sharper cognition and better clarity [in time]**
  With steadier blood sugar and a better-nourished gut microbiome, many people notice clearer thinking, improved focus and fewer of those

foggy, sluggish moments. It's a subtle shift at first, but over time it can feel like someone has gently turned the lights on in your brain.

- **More stable hormones [in time]**
  Because fibre helps regulate blood sugar and reduce inflammation, some people notice less hormonal flux. There's even some research to suggest women who eat lots of fibre have fewer menopause, PCOS and endometriosis symptoms.

- **Clearer, calmer skin [after a few months]**
  A happier gut and steadier blood sugar often show up on your face. Many notice reduced breakouts, less inflammation-driven redness and an overall brighter complexion.

- **Better weight management [ongoing]**
  Studies show that people who consistently eat more fibre tend to manage their weight better, even without focusing on calorie restriction.

- **Improved longevity and healthspan [ongoing]**
  High-fibre diets are consistently linked with living longer, healthier lives because fibre quietly supports so many systems at once: metabolic health, heart health, immunity, inflammation, cardiovascular function and even cognition. Higher-fibre diets are also linked to reduced risks of developing some cancers. Think of fibre as a daily investment that helps stack the odds in your

favour, adding not just years to your life, but life to your years.

Quiz: Are you fibre fit?

You've read about how quickly fibre can start to transform your health, now it's time to get a sense of where you're currently positioned. The following quiz offers a simple snapshot of your existing fibre habits and how well your gut might be responding. I want to be clear, it's by no means a clinical assessment, but a fun, practical tool to help you reflect on what's going well and where you might get even more benefit.

How to play

Answer the following 17 questions as honestly as you can – they'll give you a snapshot of how fibre-fit your lifestyle is right now. At the end, add up your score to work out where you're currently at and what you need to do (there's always room for improvement!) to level up your fibre intake. Consider your score as your starting point – a baseline to build on as you move through the chapters ahead.

A = 2 points

B = 1 point

C = 0 points

The Fibre-Fit Quiz

1. How often do you poo?
- **A.** 1–3 times a day
- **B.** More than 3 times a week
- **C.** Less than 3 times per week or more than 3 times a day

2. What does your poo usually look like? (Check out the Bristol Stool Chart on p. 51 – a visual aid commonly used by healthcare professionals to assess bowel health, which can also be a great tool for anyone wanting to monitor and improve their toilet habits.)
- **A.** Mostly type 3 or 4
- **B.** A mix of 2, 3, 4 and 5
- **C.** Mostly type 1, 2, 6 or 7

3. Do you suffer from constipation?
- **A.** Rarely/never
- **B.** Occasionally
- **C.** Often

4. Do you experience bloating?
- **A.** Rarely
- **B.** Sometimes (i.e. less than 3 times a week)
- **C.** Often (i.e. 3 or more times per week)

5. Do you chew your food thoroughly (i.e. 10–20 chews per bite)?
- **A.** Usually
- **B.** Sometimes
- **C.** Rarely … I tend to eat quickly

6. Do you eat sitting down and without distraction?
- **A.** Most meals
- **B.** Sometimes
- **C.** Rarely … I'm often distracted (on a device) or on the go

7. How much water do you drink each day?
- **A.** Around 2 litres or more
- **B.** 1–1.5 litres
- **C.** Less than 1 litre

8. How many different plant foods do you eat each week? (i.e. vegetables, fruit, beans, peas, chickpeas, herbs, spices, nuts and seeds)
- **A.** 30 or more
- **B.** 10–29
- **C.** Fewer than 10

9. Think about your last main meal, how many plant foods were included?
- **A.** 6 or more
- **B.** 3–5
- **C.** 2 or fewer

10. What type of bread do you usually choose?
- **A.** Wholegrain/seeded sourdough/rye
- **B.** A mix of wholegrain and white
- **C.** Mostly white bread

11. Do you eat beans, lentils and pulses?
- **A.** Most days

B. A few times (fewer than 3) per week

C. Rarely/never

12. Do you eat nuts or seeds?

A. Daily

B. A few times (fewer than 3) per week

C. Rarely/never

13. Do you choose wholegrains instead of refined grains? (i.e. wholewheat pasta, brown rice, brown bread and wholemeal flour)

A. Most of the time (more than 3 times a week)

B. Sometimes

C. Rarely

14. Do you intentionally try new fruits or vegetables?

A. Weekly

B. Occasionally

C. Rarely/never

15. Do you experience big mid-day energy crashes?

A. Rarely

B. Sometimes

C. Often

16. Do you include fermented foods in your diet? (e.g. yoghurt with live cultures, kefir, kimchi, sauerkraut, miso, tempeh or kombucha)

A. Daily or almost daily

B. A few times per week

C. Rarely/never

17. Do you regularly choose high-fibre snacks?
  A. Mostly fibre-rich choices (e.g. fruit, nuts, seeds, veg, hummus and popcorn)
  B. A mix of fibre-rich and shop-bought snacks
  C. Mostly low-fibre snacks (e.g. crisps, pastries, biscuits, chocolate bars)

Your score

0–10 points ➜ Fibre Rookie

You've got lots of room for improvement, which is exciting, because even small changes will make a huge difference to your digestion, energy and overall health.

11–24 points ➜ Fibre Explorer

You're on your way to being a Fibre Pro. Some of your habits are fibre-friendly, but there are gaps. Don't worry, the tips you'll pick up over the next few chapters are going to stack up quickly.

25–34 points ➜ Fibre Pro

You're smashing it. Your gut microbes are thriving, your digestion is probably pretty happy, and you're reaping the visible and invisible rewards of a fibre-rich lifestyle, but there's always space to optimise. I'll show you how.

How to get the most from this book

So now you're getting a glimpse of just how powerful fibre can be and hopefully starting to wonder what it could do for *you*. Let's take a look at what's to come.

The book is split into three parts, each one designed to take you a little deeper and give you practical tools you can put in place from day one, and then build on as you move through the chapters.

Part One: Unlocking the power of fibre

Here, I'll break down what fibre really is, why it matters and how it works in your body. Expect plenty of myth-busting. Carbs aren't the enemy, lectins won't ruin your life and no, you don't need to go carnivore to avoid bloating. We'll dive deeper into how fibre influences digestion, skin, hormones, mood, immunity and more. And, yes, we'll talk about poo because it's one of the best clues to what's actually going on inside your gut. I'll also give you a list of my fibre heroes and useful tips on how to shop and how to get the most from your ingredients.

Part Two: Fibre on your plate

This is where things get tasty. You'll find breakfasts, lunches, dinners and extra ideas (for things like bread, wraps and muffins) that are fibre-packed and genuinely delicious. Every recipe comes with a breakdown of the fibre content (in grams), protein (because this is still important), calories (it can be helpful to have awareness if weight loss is a goal, as I discussed in my previous book, *The 30g Plan*) and number of plants (more of this on p. 47), so you can see exactly how you're stacking things up. On pp. 221–236, you'll find meal plans and shopping lists to take the guesswork out of your week.

Part Three: Your fibre toolkit

Finally, you'll get cheat sheets, trackers and quick reference guides to make eating fibre second nature. Think charts showing fibre sources and quantities and plant diversity checklists.

The goal here isn't perfection, it's progress. Small, consistent steps add up to big wins for your digestion, energy, mood and long-term health. You'll soon see that fibre isn't boring, brown, bland ingredients like bran; it's about beautiful, colourful, mouthwatering foods that make you feel good from the inside out and that you actually look forward to eating.

It's time to unlock the full effects of fibre.

Part One

Unlocking
The Power
Of Fibre

The life-changing magic of eating more fibre

Most of us know fibre matters; few of us know just how much. This chapter shows you why it deserves your attention. We'll unpack what fibre actually is, how it teams up with your gut microbes and the impressive list of health wins it delivers. I'll introduce you to the main fibre types, explain the importance of the number 30 and show you how to spot progress in real life. Along the way, we'll see what a sample day of fibre might look like, check out some easy swaps you can make to meals and bust a few myths. No wonder I often refer to fibre as the Swiss army knife of nutrients – it really does do it all!

What *exactly* does fibre do?

Most people I work with don't give fibre a second thought, that is until they start to feel what happens when they eat more of it. Let's take a look at some of the mechanisms and benefits in more detail, so you can start to imagine the ripple effects it will have on your own health.

Energy

If you're tired of the mid-afternoon slump, fibre might be the missing piece of the puzzle. When eaten as part of a meal, soluble fibre slows the release of glucose into your system, giving you steady, sustained energy throughout the day. It does this by forming a gel in the gut that slows how quickly carbohydrates are broken down and absorbed into the bloodstream. This means glucose drips into your circulation gradually, rather than hitting all at once. Think of it as the difference between kindling and a slow-burning log: one flares up and fizzles out fast, the other keeps you going for hours. When blood sugar levels stay even, your body doesn't need to overcorrect, which can cause glucose dips that leave you fatigued and craving sugary foods.

When you feed your gut microbes fibre – their favourite food – they produce by-products called short-chain fatty acids (SCFAs) that act like little battery chargers for the cells lining your colon (colonocytes). They also lower inflammation and may even influence your metabolism, which is how your body converts food into energy. The result: more consistent energy, better focus and fewer energy crashes.

Fibre-rich foods also help stabilise hormones like insulin and GLP-1, which regulate energy balance and appetite (see more on GLP-1 on p. 20).

By the way, keep the term SCFAs in the back of your mind, as we'll be diving into it in more detail later in the chapter. These tiny compounds will continue to crop up as we peel back fibre's layers, since they're so incredibly pivotal to its health benefits.

Digestion and gut motility

When most people hear the word fibre, they instantly think of digestion. And as we've already touched on, one of fibre's most immediate effects is how it influences the movement of food through our gut. Within hours to days of increasing fibre intake, you may notice changes: smoother, easier bowel movements and more regular toilet trips.

Fibre helps to keep things moving at a comfortable pace through your gut – not too fast, not too slow – by adding bulk and softness to your poo. It also helps keep the muscles that move food through your gut gently contracting in rhythm, something known as peristalsis. This leads to a digestive system that feels more efficient, more regular and, quite simply, more in sync. But that's not all.

By keeping things moving in the gut, you become better at excreting waste, toxins, hormones (I dive into this more on p. 6), cholesterol and potentially microplastics. The beauty of increasing fibre is that you get to see the benefit every time you go to the toilet, so you can get real-life feedback on the positive impact it's having. I'll be lifting the lid on toilet habits on p. 49, and I really want to encourage poo to be less taboo.

Weight loss

Alongside a calorie deficit, fibre is perhaps one of the most underrated tools for managing weight and, refreshingly, doesn't require fad diets, hunger or injections. GLP-1 weight-loss jabs (such as Ozempic and Mounjaro) work by slowing digestion and keeping you full. Fascinatingly, fibre helps your body do this *naturally*.

When you eat fibre, your gut microbes ferment it into compounds that trigger the release of appetite-regulating hormones like GLP-1, PYY and CCK – hormones that tell your brain you've had enough to eat, steady your blood sugar and help reduce cravings. SCFAs don't just help your gut, they're also thought to support the hormones and metabolic pathways involved in how your body stores energy.

Fibre also has a clever mechanical effect. Because it adds bulk and absorbs water, it gently stretches your stomach, activating receptors that send signals to your brain to switch off hunger hormones like ghrelin. And fibre also slows the release of food from your stomach (gastric emptying), which means you feel comfortably full for longer after a fibre-filled meal.

High-fibre foods like peas, cauliflower, raspberries and broccoli do all this while providing slow, steady energy, so you can end up eating less. Eating more high-fibre, low-calorie foods – a strategy known as volume eating – can help physically fill you up. Take a look opposite for a list of high-fibre, low-calorie hero foods if you want to start volume eating for yourself.

Top 10 high-fibre, low-calorie foods

Food	Fibre (per 100g)	Calories (per 100g)
Green peas	~5.5g	~80 cals
Blackberries	~5.5g	~35 cals
Raspberries	~5g	~25 cals
Brussels sprouts	~4g	~34 cals
Broccoli	~4g	~34 cals
Carrots	~4g	~34 cals
Cauliflower	~2g	~30 cals
Spinach	~1.5g	~25 cals
Mushrooms	~1g	~7 cals
Courgettes	~0.5g	~16 cals

Skin health

Believe it or not, many scientists now believe the gut – and therefore fibre – plays a quiet but powerful role in healthy skin. Your gut and your skin are in constant conversation through what scientists call the gut–skin axis. When your gut microbes are well-fed (and remember, fibre is their favourite food!), the short-chain fatty acids they produce can help reduce inflammation throughout the body, including the skin.

Fibre also supports clear skin by keeping digestion regular and your detox pathways ticking along smoothly. A sluggish gut can allow less-than-favourable inflammatory compounds to recirculate in the body, which some preliminary studies link to acne, eczema and skin conditions such as psoriasis.

Then there's blood sugar balance. Fibre slows down the release of glucose into the bloodstream, which helps prevent insulin surges that over time can lead to advanced glycation end products (AGEs) that have been linked with the breakdown of collagen. So, from here on, think of every portion of beans, berries, oats or veg as skincare from the inside out.

Immunity

Around 70% of your immune system lives inside your gut and it's now widely thought that your gut microbes are in constant communication with this complex defence system. This means what you feed your microbes can have a considerable impact on how well your body defends itself. Fibre acts like training fuel for your immune cell army. When your gut bacteria ferment fibre, those multi-tasking short-chain fatty acids keep your gut barrier strong and selective, letting nutrients through while keeping the bad stuff like pathogens out.

This gut barrier is an important line of defence against viruses, bacteria and toxins. Think of it as a security system that decides what gets into your body and what doesn't. Fibre helps maintain the integrity of the gut barrier wall – and it's mucosal lining – so your immune system can stay calm, balanced and responsive, rather than constantly on red alert. (See the boxed section on p. 26 for more on increased intestinal permeability or 'leaky gut'.)

Fibre also supports microbial diversity, which essentially means a wide range of different bacteria species working together, and is often cited as the hallmark of a resilient immune system. Think of it like an army: the more variety you have, the better it can adapt and fight off invaders. So, whether it's the common cold or how your immune system responds to allergens, fibre quietly strengthens your defences from the inside out.

Mood

You know that 'gut feeling'? Well, it's not just a saying; there's some science behind it. Your gut and brain are in constant conversation via what's known as the gut–brain axis. Think of it as a direct phone line between your brain and your gut and the cable connecting the two is the vagus nerve.

SCFAs produced in the gut can help regulate inflammation and support the production of neurotransmitters like serotonin, dopamine and GABA, all of which play a role in mood, motivation and feeling calm and content. And, while the serotonin produced in the gut can't cross the blood-brain barrier, researchers still think that it has an influential role on levels of serotonin in the brain, even though the exact mechanism isn't fully understood yet. This was shown in the famous SMILES trial that linked a Mediterranean-style, fibre-friendly diet with significantly reduced depression scores.

Cognition and mental clarity

Fibre doesn't just influence how you feel, it also affects how clearly you think. One of the key ways it does this is by helping maintain a steady blood sugar level, which provides the brain with a consistent supply of energy. This reduces the dips that can make concentration feel harder than it should. We've already discussed the importance of a healthy gut barrier, which has also been linked with sharper cognitive function. Over time, many people notice improved mental clarity, better focus and less brain fog simply from including more fibre-rich foods in their daily routine.

Hormone regulation

Hormones are your body's chemical messengers: tiny signals that influence everything from appetite and metabolism to mood, energy, menstrual cycles and menopause symptoms. And fibre plays a surprisingly important role in keeping them functioning well.

To really understand why fibre is so powerful, particularly in women's health, we need to zoom in on the estrobolome. This is the group of microbes in your gut that help break down and recycle oestrogen and other hormones, including progesterone and testosterone. When this system is in check, excess hormones can be processed and cleared from the body smoothly. When it's not, they can recirculate, which may contribute to worse PMS, endometriosis, menopause and PCOS symptoms, as well as bloating and heavier periods. Once again, fibre quietly plays a starring role here, helping feed the microbes involved in hormone regulation and supporting the healthy elimination of them via your poo.

Fibre also supports hormone health indirectly through blood sugar regulation. When your glucose soars and crashes, your stress hormones and appetite hormones can get pulled onto the rollercoaster, too. By slowing digestion and giving you steadier energy, fibre helps keep insulin, cortisol and hunger signals like ghrelin in a healthier rhythm. The result is a body that feels more balanced and has fewer energy swings, steadier moods, better appetite signals, less hanger and, for many women, a steadier hormonal landscape through different life stages.

Reduction of long-term disease risk

Fibre isn't just about day-to-day wellbeing; it's one of the most powerful long-term health investments you can make. When researchers study populations over decades, one theme comes up again and again: the people who eat the most fibre tend to live longer, healthier lives. We're talking lower rates of type 2 diabetes, heart disease, stroke, certain cancers (particularly colorectal cancer as fibre means potentially harmful substances are removed from the body faster), fatty liver disease and metabolic syndrome. In fact, an Imperial College London analysis of nearly two million people found that every extra 10g of fibre a day was linked to around a 10% lower risk of bowel cancer.

Why? Because fibre works on so many levels at once. As we've learnt, fibre supports blood sugar control, reduces inflammation, nurtures a healthier microbiome, supports the immune system, regulates cholesterol and helps clear out waste products we no longer need. In other words, fibre creates an internal environment where disease struggles to take hold. You're stacking the odds of good overall health in your favour every time you sit down to eat. One more serving of beans, one extra handful of berries, one scoop of oats: small daily choices really do build into big, long-term benefits.

A quick word on fibre and 'leaky gut'

You may have heard the term 'leaky gut' bandied around on social media, very often with a bit of drama attached. In medical terms, it's known as increased intestinal permeability, and while it's not something most of us need to worry about, it is a real physiological process that's worth understanding.

We talked earlier about how your gut lining lets nutrients through, while keeping harmful microbes and unwanted particles out. It does this via a series of junctions that open and close like a gate. They open to let nutrients through into the bloodstream and seal tight to stop unwanted particles, such as undigested food, bacteria and irritants getting in. When the gut barrier becomes stressed or inflamed, those 'gates' can loosen. That doesn't mean your gut is full of holes, it simply means the barrier is less selective, which can nudge your immune system into overdrive and contribute to low-grade inflammation, which has been linked to everything from fatigue to autoimmune issues and allergies.

A variety of factors can influence this barrier: stress, infections, certain medications, ultra-processed diets, alcohol and, yes, not enough fibre. As we touched on earlier, short-chain fatty acids can help keep the lining strong. So, think of fibre – and the SCFAs your gut microbes produce – as daily maintenance for your gut barrier: a way of reinforcing the gut wall rather than waiting for cracks to appear.

You absolutely don't need to panic or buy expensive 'gut healing' supplements or complicated protocols. You have the most powerful tools already at your disposal: a fibre-rich diet, plenty of plant diversity, sleep, movement and stress support. Small, everyday habits really do add up and, rest assured, your gut lining is remarkably good at repairing itself when given the right conditions.

Breaking it down: What actually is fibre?

Now we know what fibre does and the benefits it brings, let's take a look at what it looks like. For far too long, fibre has been unfairly typecast as nothing more than 'roughage' – boring, bland and stuck in the shadows, while protein hogs the spotlight. Essentially, fibre is in dire need of some good PR, because it's been woefully misunderstood.

So, let's get one thing straight before we go any further: fibre is *not* the sad bowl of boring, brown bran flakes you might be picturing (although bran definitely has its place, as we'll see on p. 65 and in the recipes on pp. 122 and 212). Fibre is so much more. It's crisp apples, jewel-coloured pomegranate seeds, creamy butter beans, nutty barley flakes and rich, dark chocolate. Fibre is colourful, flavourful and physically fills you up. It brings crunch, texture and taste to the table and is anything but dull. Once you shift how you see it, fibre transforms from being the most overlooked nutrient in your kitchen cupboard to the simplest, most effective superfood you can put on your plate.

In the simplest terms, fibre is a part of carbohydrate foods that your body can't fully digest. Think of it as the scaffolding of plants: the flesh, skins, peels, seeds, stems and husks that give plants their structure. Instead of being broken down and absorbed in the small intestine, fibre passes pretty much all the way through your system more or less intact. That doesn't make it useless – far from it. In fact, it's precisely because as humans we can't digest it that fibre is so powerful.

What counts as fibre?

Ok, so we know 96% of us need to eat more fibre but what actually counts? Here's the thing, fibre is only found in plants, but it isn't one single ingredient – it's a whole family of plant compounds that share one defining trait: your body can't fully digest them. Not all fibres behave in the same way and understanding the different types will help you get the most out of them. We actually think there may be hundreds or even thousands of different types of fibre – and most plants contain a combination – but to keep things simple, let's focus on the ones that have the most research behind them.

Soluble fibre: the soother

Soluble fibre is viscous and dissolves in water to form a gel-like texture in your gut. This gel slows digestion, meaning food moves through your system at a more gradual pace. As a result, sugars are released into your bloodstream more slowly, helping to steady blood glucose levels and avoid the sharp peaks and dips that can leave you tired and hungry soon after eating.

Soluble fibre also acts like a sponge, soaking things up as it moves along your digestive tract. This is why soluble fibre – particularly a type known as beta-glucan found in oats – is often recommended to people with high LDL (the 'bad' cholesterol), because it binds to excess cholesterol in your digestive tract and helps carry it out of the body. If you're trying to reduce your LDL cholesterol, you want to be aiming for around 3g of beta-glucan a day, which might look like porridge made from 30g of rye flakes for breakfast (see p. 134), two oat cakes with your soup at lunch and 75g of pearl barley in a risotto (see p. 158) for dinner.

Insoluble fibre: the mover

Insoluble fibre is the classic 'roughage' type. Because it doesn't dissolve, it adds physical bulk to your poo and helps food move through your digestive system, keeping digestion comfortable and regular (i.e. prevents constipation).

Think of insoluble fibre as a broom, sweeping through the gut to keep everything transiting smoothly. It's found in wholegrains like bran, the outer shell of nuts and seeds, and the skins of fruit and vegetables.

Resistant starch: the hidden fibre

This one's sneaky. It's technically a type of carbohydrate that acts like prebiotic fibre (see more on this on p. 37) because it resists digestion and makes its way to your large intestine. There, it provides food for your gut microbes, something we'll discuss in detail on p. 38.

Think of resistant starch as a type of soluble fibre with special benefits. Some studies show it can increase feelings of fullness, improve insulin sensitivity and even reduce appetite. It's found in potatoes, pasta, bread and rice that have been cooked and then cooled, as well as green bananas, oats, beans and lentils. Interestingly, even if you re-heat the potatoes, pasta and rice, the resistant starch is still present. So, last night's leftover rice that you re-used today for a veggie rice dish doesn't just *taste* good, it's also *doing* you good.

Plants rarely come with just one type of fibre

While we've talked above about soluble and insoluble fibre separately, nature doesn't always deliver them in neat little boxes. Most plants contain a blend of fibres that work together, synergistically in your gut.

Think of a bean: the outer skin is mostly insoluble fibre, helping add bulk and keeping digestion moving, while the soft inside is rich in soluble fibre that supports digestion. Asparagus works the same way: the fibrous tips and stems provide insoluble fibre, while the tender flesh offers soluble fibre.

This combination is part of why whole plant foods are so powerful and why you don't have to overly fixate on chasing specific fibre types. By simply incorporating a variety of plants in your diet, you naturally get a balance of the various health-promoting fibres.

Types of fibre (at a glance)

Fibre type	Found in	Why it helps
Pectin	Apples, pears, berries, citrus	Steadies blood sugar; supports cholesterol; feeds good microbes
Beta-glucan	Oats, oat bran, barley	Lowers LDL cholesterol; improves blood sugar; increases fullness
Inulin/FOS	Onions, garlic, leeks, asparagus, chicory	Prebiotic; boosts beneficial bacteria; supports gut lining
GOS	Dairy, legumes, live yoghurts	Feeds the good bacteria, Bifidobacteria; supports digestion; may ease IBS symptoms
Resistant starch	Cooked and cooled potatoes/rice/pasta, green bananas, oats, legumes	Feeds butyrate producers; supports gut barrier; improves insulin response
Cellulose	Veg, fruit skins, nuts, seeds, wholegrains	Adds bulk to poo; supports regularity
Lignin	Flaxseeds, sesame seeds, wholegrains	Supports bowel function; has antioxidant effects
Mucilage	Okra, chia seeds, flaxseeds, basil seeds, psyllium husk	Helps poo form and pass easily

The gut microbiome (and why fibre is its favourite food)

This is a book about fibre so I don't want to go too deep into gut health, but we can't talk about fibre without mentioning the microbiome. Inside your gut (in your large intestine mostly) lives a bustling ecosystem of microbes – good bacteria, yeasts, viruses (the helpful kind!) and fungi – all working round the clock to help you digest food, synthesise vitamins like B12 and K2, defend against disease and stay healthy.

I like to think of the large intestine (otherwise known as the colon) as a community garden: you provide the plot and the fertiliser; your microbes do the germinating and cultivating. When the garden is diverse and well-fed, everything flourishes. When it's starved of food (fibre), it can become overrun by weeds and get a bit out of control (dysbiosis).

Here's the crucial bit: your gut microbes' staple fuel is fibre – specifically, a type of fibre called prebiotic fibre (which I'll guide you through later). When prebiotic fibre arrives in the colon, your microbes set about breaking it down through a process known as fermentation. From that process they make a cocktail of powerful compounds – short-chain fatty acids (SCFAs), which we have met a number of times already in the 'What *exactly* does fibre do?' section – that support gut integrity, calm inflammation, talk to hormones and send 'all is well' signals throughout your body.

What your gut microbes do

1. **Influence your mental wellbeing.** Your microbes are constantly communicating with your brain via the vagus nerve, which, as you'll remember from p. 23, acts like a phone line linking the brain and gut.

2. **Fortify your gut lining.** As discussed on p. 22, a well-fed microbiome helps maintain a strong, selective gut barrier, letting beneficial nutrients in and keeping harmful irritants out.

3. **Train your immune system.** 70% of your immune system is located in the gut, and microbes are in constant conversation with the immune cells that line the gut. When well-fed on fibre, microbes help your immune army stay steady and discerning rather than jumpy and overreactive.

4. **Help with metabolism and appetite rhythms.** SCFAs talk to the hormones that influence fullness, blood sugar steadiness and energy.

5. **Support microbial diversity.** Different plants bring different fibres; different fibres feed different species. And different microbe species all have different benefits – Akkermansia, for example, is a bacteria known for enhancing insulin sensitivity (see the box on pp. 36–7 for more species). Variety on your plate equates to variety in your microbiome, which is linked with better health outcomes overall. Lower levels of gut microbe diversity can potentially increase the risk of developing conditions such as inflammatory bowel disease, eczema and type 2 diabetes.

Why fibre changes everything

Because fibre is your microbes' main food source, eating more of it changes *who* thrives in your gut and *what* they produce. Over time, this positively influences your digestion, energy, mood and immunity. Think of it less like planting a single type of seed on some terrain (your gut) and more like rewilding it: you want small, consistent inputs – in the form of lots of different plants – to restore and maintain variety and balance.

Two principles to hold in mind:

1. **Diversity beats perfection.** No single 'super fibre' wins; we're looking for a mix of plants to grow a resilient inner ecosystem.

2. **Dose makes the difference.** If you're not used to much fibre, your microbes need a training plan. Later, in Chapter 3, you'll learn the importance of introducing more fibre into your diet gradually, so you get all the benefits without side-effects like bloating and wind.

The microbiome decoded

Microbiome: The whole gut ecosystem that contains your gut microbes, plus their genes and the environment they live in. Think of it as the entire 'microbial world' inside your gut.

Microbiota: The actual organisms themselves: the bacteria, viruses, fungi and other microbes living in your gut. They're the residents; the microbiome is their neighbourhood and your microbiota are completely unique to you. Diet, medications, genetics, your age, where you live, how you were born (i.e. vaginal delivery or Caesarean) and even your pets all play a role in the make-up of your gut microbiome.

Fermentation: The process undertaken by microbes when they eat (break down) fibre and turn it into helpful compounds (short-chain fatty acids).

Short-chain fatty acids (SCFAs): Powerful compounds your gut microbes make when they ferment fibre. The main ones are butyrate, acetate and propionate (see below and p.36). They help strengthen your gut lining, calm inflammation, support immunity and even influence energy, mental health and mood. They're one of the main reasons fibre is such a hero nutrient.

Butyrate: Linked to a stronger and more resilient gut barrier, less inflammation – especially important for people with conditions such as irritable bowel syndrome (IBS), ulcerative colitis and Crohn's disease – and even potentially increased glucose control, blood pressure regulation and insulin sensitivity.

Acetate: The most abundant short-chain fatty acid, helping provide fuel for many cells in the body, supporting appetite regulation and helping maintain the right pH in the gut for beneficial microbes to thrive. It's the crowd-pleaser of the SCFA family – widely used, widely helpful.

Propionate: A short-chain fatty acid that travels to the liver, where it helps regulate cholesterol production and glucose metabolism. It also plays a role in appetite signalling and so can help you feel satisfied after eating.

Gut barrier: The microscopic (it's only one cell thick) lining of your gut that acts like a gate, letting nutrients through to the bloodstream and keeping trouble out.

Diversity: This means having a wide variety of different microbes in your gut. Each species has its own role, so a diverse gut microbiome generally translates to a stronger and more efficient workforce. Different fibres feed different microbes, which is why a varied plant-rich diet helps grow a stronger, more balanced microbiome. There are some 38 trillion bacteria in your gut – made up of different families and species – and we're merely brushing the surface when it comes to understanding them.

Lentils boost *Faecalibacterium*, a major butyrate producer.

Peas feed *Bifidobacteria*, linked to lower inflammation.

Broad beans increase *Akkermansia*, related to metabolic health.

Meet the biotics

Now you have a better understanding of the microbiome and the roles that different microbes play, the next step is to look at what actually influences them. That's where the 'biotics' come in – the fibres, live bacteria and microbial metabolites (i.e. by-products) that help your gut ecosystem thrive.

You've probably seen the words prebiotic and probiotic splashed across yoghurt pots or supplement labels. You may even have come across the less common terms postbiotic and synbiotic and wondered whether it's all a clever marketing ruse? Spoiler: it's not (at least not always). There's real science here and it's fascinating.

Let's break down who's who in this epic soap opera that's flourishing inside your gut.

Prebiotics

I touched on prebiotic fibre already on p. 32 but it plays such an important role that I want to delve into it a little deeper here. You'll probably remember that prebiotics are types of soluble fibre that your body can't digest, but your microbes absolutely love. If we continue the analogy of your gut as a thriving garden, then prebiotics are the fertiliser that feeds the soil so the flowers (your good bacteria) can bloom.

Prebiotics are found naturally in a whole host of plant foods but particularly in things like onions, garlic, leeks, asparagus, oats, apples and bananas. Remember when we talked about the cooled potatoes or rice from last night's dinner containing something called resistant starch? Well, this is also considered a prebiotic.

Within the prebiotic family, there are a number of different types. Each one works in a slightly different way to support your gut health. You don't need to know them inside out, but it helps to understand what they do and where they come from.

Inulin *(found in chicory root, Jerusalem artichokes, leeks, asparagus, onions and garlic)*

Inulin is a powerful fermentable fibre that's especially good at feeding *Bifidobacteria* – the friendly microbes linked to improved immune health. It's naturally slightly sweet and a concentrated form can be extracted from plants and processed into a powder to boost fibre in foods.

Fructooligosaccharides (FOS) *(found in fruits and vegetables, especially green bananas, onions and asparagus)*

FOS are easily fermented by gut bacteria and help increase beneficial microbes. They also work gently to support regular bowel movements.

Galactooligosaccharides (GOS) *(found in dairy products and also added to some yoghurts and baby formulas)*

GOS are especially good at feeding bifidobacteria and are often used to support gut health in babies and adults alike. They can help reduce bloating and support a balanced microbiome.

Polyphenols *(antioxidant compounds found in the skins of richly coloured fruits and vegetables, as well as in spices and herbs)* and **omega-3s** *(found in oily fish)* are also considered prebiotics and provide food for your gut microbes, so definitely worth including in your diet. Think blueberries, aubergines, black beans, oregano and cinnamon for polyphenols. And salmon, sardines, mackerel, flaxseeds, walnuts and chia seeds for omega 3. I'll guide you through more about polyphenols on p. 47.

Probiotics

These are live, beneficial bacteria that join your gut's existing population to help keep things balanced and resilient. You'll find probiotics in fermented foods like yoghurt, kefir, kimchi, sauerkraut, miso and kombucha, all created by friendly microbes doing their natural fermentation magic. That tangy flavour? That's a sign they're alive and kicking. Speaking of which, the oldest known woman in the world – Maria Branyas Morera – who lived to 117, ate three yoghurts a day. Obviously, we don't know the exact reason for her long life but I'd like to think her consumption of live bacteria helped!

Interestingly, the act of heating foods can kill off probiotics – this occurs in the case of baking a loaf of sourdough, for example – but scientists still think that even dead probiotics may have beneficial health properties. Great news for bread fans!

Think of probiotics as temporary houseguests: some move in for a short stay and leave after doing their job, while others may stick around longer if the environment (your gut) is welcoming.

Not all probiotics do the same thing. Some strains are great at calming inflammation, others excel at restoring balance after antibiotics, and some have links to mental well being. People often notice subtle but meaningful changes when live bacteria from probiotics become a habit. Think better digestion, less bloating after meals and even improved skin. And if you're thinking, 'Well, I'll just pop some probiotic supplements,' you might want to skip to p. 87 for the full lowdown on when they're useful and when they're not, and why food is often better.

Synbiotics

What happens when you put prebiotics and probiotics together? Enter synbiotics: the dynamic duo of gut health that work together synergistically to make sure the live bacteria you eat (probiotics) have the food they need to thrive (prebiotics), potentially leading to a more balanced and diverse gut microbiome.

You can find synbiotics in certain yoghurts, fortified drinks or supplements. But you can also create a synbiotic meal at home incredibly easily and without trying too hard. A great example is a bowl of overnight oats made with live yoghurt (the probiotic) and oats, chia seeds and berries (the prebiotics).

Postbiotics

Here's where the real magic happens. Postbiotics are the beneficial substances created by your gut microbes when they digest prebiotics. Think of them as the handwritten thank-you notes your gut microbes send you for feeding them well.

The stars of the show are the SCFAs butyrate, acetate and propionate (which we met on pp. 35–36). They nourish the cells lining your colon, keep inflammation in check, and even influence your mood and brain function. Some scientists call them the peace-keepers of the gut.

It's wild to think your gut microbes take fibre – something you can't digest – and turn it into compounds that fuel your body and brain. That's fibre alchemy at its finest. So, when we talk about eating fibre for gut health, what we really mean is eating to source and produce more of these postbiotic goodies.

The 'biotics' at a glance

	What is it?	Where do you find it?	What does it do?
Prebiotics	Soluble fibre that feeds your gut microbes	Garlic, onions, oats, bananas, asparagus	Nourishes good bacteria; supports digestion
Probiotics	Live 'good' bacteria	Fermented foods, e.g. yoghurt, kefir, kimchi, sauerkraut	Adds balance, aids immunity, supports mood
Synbiotics	Prebiotics + probiotics working together	Yoghurt + oats + seeds + berries; miso soup + leeks + onions	Enhances overall gut health synergy
Postbiotics	Compounds made by your gut microbes	Produced inside your gut	Strengthens gut lining and reduces inflammation

When you see how these 'biotics' interconnect, you realise fibre is at the heart of a big, beautiful complex system that affects everything from digestion to energy and even emotions. It's the quiet multi-tasker that helps your gut ecosystem thrive. And, while I've run you through the key players above, I don't want you to get too bogged down in the minutiae of all the different types of fibre and trying to formulate meals that include all of them. As you'll see as we head through the next couple of chapters, the real key is simply to make sure you're getting close to 30g of fibre each day and to get that fibre from as many different plant sources as possible. From here on, diversity should be your number one fibre goal and your new mantra.

How much fibre do I need?

We know from studies that 30g a day is the baseline of how much fibre you should be aiming for to reap all the health benefits we've discussed. Currently in the UK, most of us are only hitting 18g a day. In the US it's more like 15g. It's worth repeating that in the UK, 96% of us are not reaching the recommended daily amount and women generally consume less fibre than men.

Clearly, we have a long way to go collectively, but, don't despair, because now you have this book in your hands you'll find it's really not that hard, once you put your mind to it. And if you're one of the few people actually nailing the 30g target (take a look opposite to see what this might look like) hats off to you, but there's still more you can do. What we see from the studies is that health benefits incrementally stack up even further beyond the 30g threshold, so when it comes to fibre, more – both in terms of quantity and diversity – really is more. Of course, we also want to be making sure that we're consuming protein and healthy fats alongside all this wonderful fibre, which I have included in the recipes in Part Two.

Here's a sample day showing you how eating 30g of fibre might look:

Breakfast

Greek yoghurt bowl with berries, flaxseeds and chia = 14g fibre

- 150g Greek yoghurt (0g)
- 80g raspberries (3g)
- 1 tbsp chia seeds (5g)
- 1 tbsp ground flaxseeds (4g)
- Small handful of mixed nuts (2g)

Lunch

Wholegrain wrap with hummus, egg and avocado = 11g fibre

- 1 wholegrain tortilla wrap (6g)
- 1 egg (0g)
- 1 heaped tbsp hummus (3g)
- ½ small avocado (2g)

Snack

1 medium apple (1g)

Dinner

Stir-fry veg with tofu = 7g

- ½ pack (125g) stir-fry veg (5g)
- ⅓ block (75g) tofu (0.5g)
- ½ pouch (125g) of cooked brown rice (1g)
- 1 tsp sesame seeds (0.5g)

Total ≈ 32g fibre

The Tanzanian Hadza tribes – often cited as having one of the most diverse microbiomes in the world – regularly hit over 100g fibre a day and have the lowest incidence of chronic disease in the world. That doesn't mean *you* need to aim that high – trust me, it would probably come with a lot of gastrointestinal discomfort if you weren't used to it – but have it in the back of your mind that the health benefits of fibre don't stop at 30g. One large study in the *American Journal of Epidemiology* found that for every extra 10g of fibre eaten per day, people had around a 10% lower risk of dying from any cause during the study period. Put simply: more fibre was linked with a longer, healthier life.

Want to know what an extra 10g of fibre in your diet might look like look in real life? Take a look below or simply stack two of the '5g of fibre' examples I've included on p. 102.

Easy ways to add an extra 10g into your day:

- 1 tbsp chia seeds added to your overnight oats at breakfast + half an avocado with your sandwich at lunch
- 1 slice rye toast with crunchy peanut butter for breakfast + 100g legume pasta for dinner
- ½ tin chickpeas with your salad at lunch + handful raspberries with your dessert
- 1 generous cupped handful of broccoli + 1 medium (120g) roasted sweet potato at dinner

- 150g roasted edamame beans as a topper on your soup
- 40g air-popped popcorn + an apple + 20 almonds as a snack

Think 30:30

Ok, we've covered a fair bit of science and, having possibly introduced you to a number of new concepts, you may well be feeling a little overwhelmed. Understandable! On one level, fibre is a simple concept, but when you delve deeply into all its layers, it can start to feel quite complicated.

One of my key missions is to simplify nutrition as much as possible, so let's strip the fibre chat right back. When in doubt about what and how much fibre to eat, just remember 30:30. It's a simple guide to help you on your way to eating enough fibre and enough variety. Let's take a quick look at why:

30g of fibre a day

We've already explored why fibre matters and we know that the UK government recommendation is a minimum of 30g a day. This guideline was established by SACN (the Scientific Advisory Committee for Nutrition) after reviewing studies that linked higher fibre intake with a protective effect on health, from lowering heart disease risk to helping manage weight – go back to p. 17 for a reminder of the full list of fibre benefits.

30 different plants a week

Each plant has its own unique fibres and other prebiotic plant compounds, like polyphenols, which selectively feed different species of gut bacteria. The more variety of plants you eat, the richer and more resilient your microbial community becomes and the more likely they are to reward you with SCFAs. The American Gut Project's research in 2018 – which looked at the eating habits of over 10,000 people – demonstrated that those with the healthiest (i.e. most diverse) gut microbiotas ate thirty or more different plant types a week. And to be clear, when we talk about 'plants', we're talking about fruit, vegetables, legumes (chickpeas, lentils, beans), nuts, seeds *and* herbs and spices. Hence why many nutrition scientists recommend 'eating the rainbow' – a perfect excuse to load up on brightly hued berries, dark green leafy veg and vibrant spices like turmeric and paprika.

It's important to note that different-coloured fruit and veg from the same family count as separate plants, so when you're at your local grocer's look out for yellow and purple carrots, purple sprouting broccoli and Romanesco cauliflower – the range of colours denote different polyphenols, which all confer their own health benefits. Even olive oil, dark chocolate, tea and coffee have been shown to have beneficial plant chemicals. See the plant diversity wheel on p. 243 for more inspiration.

One way to ensure you're getting a wide range of plants is to track them – giving yourself 1 point for every unique plant eaten across the course of a week. I've included plant points in all the recipes, as well as a plant tracker template that might be fun to fill in on p. 244 (though, of course, you could equally just note down the different plants as you eat them on your phone or in a journal). It's a great way to motivate yourself and your friends and family if you wanted to make it into a challenge. It can also be the nudge you need to try new recipes and ingredients now and then. Of course, you don't need to track obsessively, this is a fun reminder to eat a more varied diet, not something you need to feel pressured to do day in, day out.

The benefits of eating the rainbow

Colour/ Polyphenol Type	Found in	Why it helps
Red – Lycopene/ Anthocyanins	Tomatoes, watermelon, strawberries, papaya	Antioxidant; may reduce cancer risk; supports heart health
Orange – Carotenoids	Carrots, sweet potatoes, apricots, orange peppers	Eye health; immune support
Yellow – Flavonoids	Yellow peppers, pineapple, mango, lemons	Anti-inflammatory; supports immunity
Green – Catechins /Flavones	Spinach, kale, broccoli, kiwi, green tea	Antioxidant; supports gut and immune health
Blue/Purple – Anthocyanins/ Resveratrol	Blueberries, blackberries, grapes, aubergine	Brain and heart health
Brown – Flavanols /Phenolic acids	Coffee, cocoa, dark chocolate, wholegrains	Supports microbiome; metabolic benefits
White – Allicin/ Flavanols	Garlic, onions, mushrooms, cauliflower	Antimicrobial; supports heart health

A quick note on plant points

Some nutritionists follow a strict plant points system, whereby each unique plant eaten gets you one point but some – like spices, herbs and olive oil – are only worth a quarter of a point. This is just too convoluted for me. I want to make healthy eating easier, not more exhausting. Plus remember, this isn't an exact science – the research was based on observational studies, which don't prove cause and effect. So don't stress over half and quarter points, just know it's all adding up. And rest assured that all the recipes in Part Two don't just meet this target, but go far beyond it. You'll find the number of unique plants listed in each of the recipes, but I haven't included olive oil in the totals (though it does have impressive levels of polyphenols, which your gut microbes love). You'll be pleased to know dark chocolate, legume pasta and different-coloured types of the same food (e.g. peppers) all count as a unique plant.

How do I know if it's working?

Making poo less taboo

Forget expensive – and often unsubstantiated – gut health tests. What you see in the toilet bowl is one of the best clues to what's happening inside your gut. The colour, shape and consistency of your poo offers real-time feedback on how well your digestion and your fibre are working together. Here's a quick guide to what's normal, what's not and when to get checked out.

What's normal

- **Frequency:** Anywhere from 3 times a day to 3 times a week is the medical definition of 'normal', but we're all unique and so your normal toilet habits might look slightly different. If you poo 4 times a day and always have since you can remember, there's probably no need to worry.
- **Effortless:** You should go to the toilet easily with no straining. It can sometimes help to raise your feet so that your knees are higher than your hips. You can buy special 'squatty potty' stools for this, although just using a small bathroom bin if you have one handy or a couple of spare toilet rolls under each foot can be equally effective.

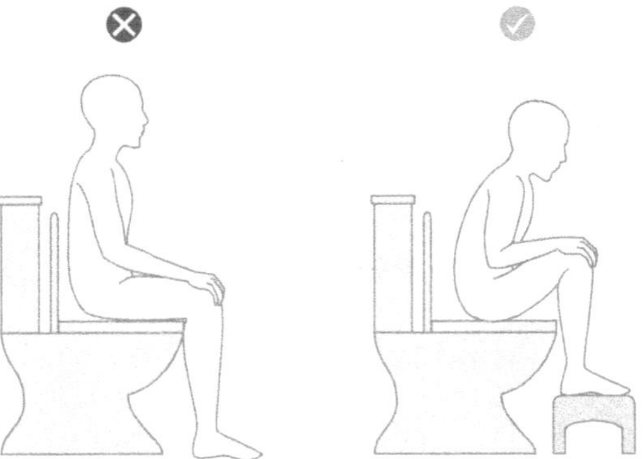

- **No urgency:** You should have good control over your bowel – no running to the toilet or having near misses.
- **Shape:** Think Bristol Stool Chart types 3–4: smooth or softly formed.

BRISTOL STOOL CHART

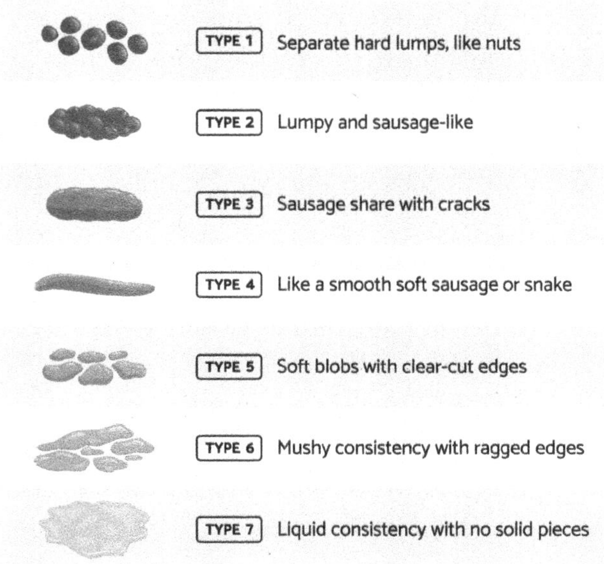

- **Gut transit time:** The time that food takes to pass through (and out) of your body can be anywhere between 10 and 72 hours, with 24–36 hours being the average. Interestingly, women can be at the higher end due to them having a longer colon (about 15cm more) than men. Progesterone can also slow things down, so women may find their digestion is more sluggish in the second half of their cycle and especially during pregnancy. A very crude way of testing your transit time is to eat sweetcorn kernels and see how long takes to see them come out in your poo.

- **Colour:** A mid-brown is ideal and is due to a mix of bile and bilirubin. Dark poo can be a sign of blood and needs to be checked out by your GP, but can also be related to your diet (beetroot is a common culprit!) or medications such as iron supplements.
- **'Ghost wipes':** Clean paper with no residue after wiping can be a sign that you've fully evacuated.

When it's worth a second look

- Bloody, black, pale, mucus or oily poos that are hard to flush.
- Sticky poo isn't usually a cause for concern if it's occasional – it can be a sign of dehydration, not enough fibre or too much dietary fat – but should be investigated if persistent.
- A sudden or persistent change in bowel habit (especially if it lasts more than three weeks).
- Feeling like you haven't fully evacuated everything out.
- Waking at night to poo.
- Unintentional weight loss, fatigue or anaemia.
- Abdominal pain or persistent bloating (even when you wake up in the morning).

Please see your doctor if any of these apply.

About farts

- 10–20 a day is absolutely normal, honest! And most of us expel around 600ml gas across the day, but some people produce much more.

- Farts come from fibre fermentation and is a sign your microbes are busy.
- Strong odour can come from an increase in sulphur-containing foods, like onions, garlic, eggs, broccoli and cabbage. It can also be due to too much protein and not enough fibre.
- Extreme bloating, pain or persistent offensive smell should be discussed with your doctor.

Don't waste money on ...

- **Microbiome tests:** The data may look clever, but it isn't clinically useful (yet). This may change in the future as we learn more about what bacteria species actually make up an optimal microbiome profile, but currently we just don't have this kind of intelligence for humans. What we do know is that pretty much every single one of us could benefit from eating more fibre!
- **Activated charcoal supplements:** These can interfere with the absorption of medications. They are used in medical settings in case of overdoses and poisoning, so leave it to the doctors to decide whether it's needed and stay away from home remedies.
- **Gut 'cleanses' or 'detox teas':** They don't remove toxins; your liver and gut already do that beautifully.
- **Colonics:** Despite big detox claims, there's no evidence showing these improve gut health or remove toxins, and can actually disrupt your natural microbiome.

Fibre FAQs: Sorting facts from fear

Fibre can seem complicated with all the conflicting advice out there. Let's clear the confusion, bust some myths and look at practical tips to make fibre part of your everyday life, without overthinking it.

1. Fibre is found in carbs, but aren't carbs bad for you?

Carbohydrates have a bad reputation, but not all carbs are created equal and they are certainly not the enemy. In fact, many of the most nourishing, gut-supportive foods available to us are carbohydrates.

Many people hear the word carbs and immediately think of biscuits, bread, chips, pizza and pastries. Society seems to have bundled all carbs into one box and labelled them 'bad'. Whereas, actually, they're an incredibly diverse group and lumping them all together misses the point.

The carbs that support our health look very different: oats, rice, beans, lentils, vegetables, fruit. These foods are naturally rich in fibre, packed with vitamins, minerals and powerful plant compounds and play a vital role in nourishing our gut. So, instead of cutting out carbs, think about preferentially choosing ones that come from whole plants, rather than packets. Following a low-carb diet is going to make it pretty much impossible to hit the 30g target and is just one of the reasons I don't recommend this way of eating.

2. Do lectins or phytates negate the benefits of fibre?

Lectins and phytates are natural compounds in beans, nuts and wholegrains. Yes, they can slightly reduce mineral absorption, but normal amounts are perfectly safe. Cooking, soaking or fermenting reduces them. The fibre and nutrients you get far outweigh any tiny downsides, so no need to worry about them.

3. Supplements: yes or no?

Most people can reach fibre targets through food first: beans, lentils, wholegrains, fruit, veg, nuts and seeds (see Chapter 2 for our fibre heroes). Supplements like psyllium or inulin can help if your diet is low in fibre, but whole foods bring extra vitamins, minerals and phytonutrients, which play their own important roles in health. I dive into supplements more on page 86.

4. How does fibre look in a low-carb keto or carnivore diet?

Although research in this area is quite limited, strict keto and carnivore diets are very low in fibre and can affect gut diversity, with some studies suggesting a loss in certain beneficial bacterial species, such as bifidobacteria. Even small amounts of vegetables, nuts or seeds can help maintain a healthier microbiome but, ideally, we should all be aiming for at least 30g of fibre a day – see a sample day on page 44.

If you're a fan of meat, fish and dairy, don't worry, no one is saying you have to give them up. Eating your thirty different plants a week alongside your favourite meals means you'll be maximising your health, but not missing out on the foods you love. And, of course, meat, fish and dairy have lots of other benefits, such as protein, which are not covered in depth here, but which I do discuss at length in my previous book, *The 30g Plan*.

It's worth pointing out that a diet that's high in animal products and/or ultra-processed foods is more likely to promote a less-favourable gut microbiome. This is just one of the reasons I don't promote a carnivore or strict keto way of eating, especially as a 2014 study in *Nature* journal showed an increase in bacteria associated with inflammatory bowel disease in people following a carnivore diet after just five days.

5. Is gluten-free better for fibre?

Many gluten-free processed foods are lower in fibre than wheat-based options and studies have shown that people who avoid gluten often have reduce microbial diversity in their gut flora (their microbiota). If you really can't tolerate gluten or are coeliac, focus on including plenty of naturally gluten-free whole foods in your diet, like brown rice, quinoa, millet, buckwheat, corn, legumes, vegetables and fruit for fibre. Oats are naturally gluten-free but are often processed in factories that also handle gluten-containing foods, so if you are avoiding gluten, it's worth actively seeking out oat brands that assure they're not cross-contaminated (check the labels).

6. Can too much fibre be harmful?

It's true that sudden increases in fibre can cause bloating, gas or discomfort, so the key is to increase your fibre intake gradually and drink plenty of water to encourage it to move through your gut. Build up slowly if you're currently on the low side of the recommended 30g. Check out page 57 for a deep dive into this important topic.

7. How much fibre do my kids need?

Fibre is important for kids, too, but once again the statistics are not looking good. The National Diet and Nutrition Survey reports that 78% of kids aged 18 months to 3 years, and 86% of those aged 4–10 years aren't meeting recommended amounts.

According to the NHS, toddlers (2–3 years) need ~15g/day and older children and teens ~25g/day. For a more detailed target, take your kid's age in years and add 5g.

Here's a quick reference guide:

Age	Fibre target (grams/day)
2–5 years	15g
5–11 years	20g
11–16 years	25g
16+ years	30g

A day of eating for a toddler might look something like this. Don't worry if your child eats more – this is just an idea of how much is needed to reach the recommended 15g:

Breakfast

Porridge with fruit

- 3 tbsp porridge oats cooked with milk (2g)
- Handful of mashed raspberries (2g)
- Sprinkle of chopped walnuts (1g)

Total: 5g fibre

Lunch

- ½ multi-seed bagel (2g)
- 1 tbsp hummus (1.5g)
- 2.5cm chunk cucumber (0.5g)

Total: 4g fibre

Dinner

Spaghetti bolognese

- 40g wholewheat pasta (5g)
- Minced beef (0g)
- 2 tbsp peas (2g)

Total: 7g

Daily total: 16g fibre

8. I heard fibre isn't essential and we can live without it.

Yes, strictly speaking that's true, but it's the equivalent of saying you can survive without exercise. Surviving and thriving are very different beasts. When gut bacteria are deprived of fibre, they can start to eat and break down the gut lining, which negatively impacts the gut barrier. It also has downstream consequences on metabolic health, immune health and gut-brain health, as well as increasing the risk of colon cancer. Not eating enough fibre can also just make you feel more sluggish and less sharp and can impact your skin – as we've already discussed. Eating more fibre is also associated with a longer (and healthier) life, which is probably the biggest reason of all to eat more of it.

9. How can I track how much fibre I'm eating?

There are some great apps to help with this. I personally like @nutracheck, but there's also @cronometer and @myfitnesspal, which also track other nutrients such as protein, as well as calories if that's of interest. It's important to note that these apps aren't a hundred per cent accurate, so look on them as a handy guide rather than absolute gospel truth.

10. Can I get fibre from drinks?

Smoothies count if they include whole fruit, veg or oats. Juices without pulp unfortunately don't contribute any meaningful fibre. There are lots of prebiotic soft drinks with added fibre hitting the market now. While they can be a convenient way to incorporate more fibre into your diet, I wouldn't rely only on them (especially if they have lots of added sugars). It's more important to reach your fibre goals through whole foods where possible.

11. Why do women tend to be more prone to gut health issues like constipation than men?

Women are more prone to constipation and gut discomfort than men for a few key reasons, many of them hormonal. Fluctuations in oestrogen and progesterone across the menstrual cycle can affect motility, i.e. how quickly the gut moves. For example, progesterone rises in the second half of the cycle and can slow down bowel movements, making constipation more likely in the lead-up to menstruation. During pregnancy, these hormonal shifts are even stronger, which is why constipation is so common.

Women also tend to have a slightly longer colon (up to 15cm more!) and more twists and loops, which can contribute to bloating and sluggish digestion. Pelvic floor differences may play a role, too: pregnancy and childbirth can affect the muscles involved in pushing out a poo – just one more very important reason to do your pelvic floor exercises.

A quick recap

Fibre isn't just about keeping things moving, it's the quiet powerhouse behind good gut health, balanced hormones, stable energy and a calm, resilient mood. Once you see how it works, it's impossible not to fall a little bit in love with fibre.

- Fibre is the part of plants that your body can't fully digest, but your gut microbes can, and they turn it into beneficial by-products.

- Those by-products are called short-chain fatty acids (SCFAs), they protect your gut, balance inflammation and boost immunity.

- Most of us consume just 18g of fibre a day, which is far short of the recommended 30g.

- Not all fibre is the same:
  - » **Soluble** (think oats, apples, beans)
  - » **Insoluble** (wholegrains, skins, seeds)
  - » **Resistant starch** (cooked and cooled potatoes, bread that's frozen then toasted)
  - » **Prebiotic fibres** feed your gut microbes (onions, garlic, leeks)

Although this last point is interesting, please don't worry too much about the different types, the key is to aim for getting enough and from as many different types of plants as possible.

Next up, in Chapter 2, we'll look at 'fibre heroes': the best everyday sources of fibre, their benefits and easy ways to incorporate them into your diet.

CHAPTER 2

Your fibre roadmap

So, now you know *why* fibre matters, let's talk about the foods that make hitting your fibre goals feel joyful, delicious and effortless. You see, not all plants pull equal weight in the fibre department; the best ones deliver fibre plus a whole package of nutrients, prebiotics, antioxidants and gut-loving goodness. Think of this chapter as your VIP tour of the plant world's overachievers: the everyday ingredients that can transform your meals, your microbiome and the way you feel, without having to overhaul your entire diet. Let's meet the fibre stars that deserve a regular place on your plate.

Fibre heroes

We know that fibre comes from plants – fruit, veg, nuts, seeds, legumes and wholegrains – but there are definitely some sources that pack more nutrient punch than others. Think of these as your fibre heroes: the ingredients that do double (and sometimes triple) the hard graft.

These ingredients don't just boost your fibre intake, they bring along vitamins, minerals, polyphenols and other plant compounds that support your gut, balance your blood sugar and keep your immune system humming. From humble lentils and oats to chia seeds, berries and broccoli, each one has a superpower – whether it's feeding your gut microbes, lowering cholesterol or keeping digestion moving. In this section, we'll meet the standout stars worthy of a regular spot on your plate, learn what makes them special and find easy ways to build them into your everyday meals.

Oats

If there's one fibre hero worth a permanent spot on your breakfast table, it's oats, with just two tablespoons providing 2.5g of fibre. Their secret weapon is beta-glucan, a soluble fibre that forms a gel in your gut, helping to slow digestion, steady blood sugar and lower LDL cholesterol. Think of it as your digestion's slow-release brake keeping things moving at just the right pace so your energy stays smooth and steady, rather than peaking and crashing.

Beta-glucan also feeds your beneficial gut bacteria, helping them produce those short-chain fatty acids that help quash inflammation and keep your gut lining strong. And because oats digest slowly, they keep you fuller for longer.

Oats are also versatile and affordable. From overnight oats to porridge, breakfast bakes and smoothies, they're one of the simplest ways to add fibre to your day. For an extra gut-loving boost, try pairing oats with yoghurt (for probiotics) and berries (for polyphenols and extra fibre): a delicious synbiotic breakfast that your microbiome will thank you for – take a look at Salted caramel overnight oats on p. 136 and Cherry bakewell overnight oats on p. 125 for inspiration.

Wheat bran

This is classic 'roughage' – the outer layer of the wheat kernel that gives your gut a gentle workout. It's rich in insoluble fibre, so adds bulk to your poo – making it easier to push it out – and supports regularity. It doesn't really taste of anything, if I'm being honest, but is a great way to boost texture and crunch in porridge, overnight oats, baked goods and homemade granola.

Start small if you're new to it, it's pretty potent stuff – over 40g of fibre per 100g – and best introduced gradually. A tablespoon stirred into porridge or yoghurt can transform your breakfast into a fibre-rich powerhouse. You'll find wheat bran in the Soaked pearl barley porridge on p. 122 and in some of the chia pudding recipes on p. 128.

Oat bran

Oat bran is the outer layer of the oat grain, which gives it almost double the fibre of regular porridge oats. It's rich in beta-glucans, which is the type of fibre that's been shown to help lower cholesterol. Oat bran flakes are smaller in size than other oats, which gives a creamy texture to porridge or smoothies and works well in baking (check out the Apple and raspberry buckwheat muffins on p. 208). Oat bran has 4g fibre per 30g serving, compared to regular oats, which have 2.3g per 30g.

I use oat bran interchangeably with regular oats, mostly in porridge, overnight oats and baking, and have included it in the Healthier oat bran cookies on p. 212. Do be aware that because it's smaller in size, it cooks faster (about half the time) than regular oats when making porridge.

Chickpeas

If oats are your slow-release brake, chickpeas are your gut's multitaskers. Packed with both soluble and insoluble fibre, they help feed your beneficial gut microbes *and* keep everything moving smoothly through your digestive tract. That combination makes them brilliant for digestion, satiety and blood sugar balance all at once. Chickpeas also contain resistant starch (which we talked about on page 30) that acts like fibre because it resists digestion and goes straight to your large intestine, where your microbes feast on it.

From sandwich fillings (see Crushed chickpea-stuffed pitta p. 143) to tray bakes (Chicken, chickpea and feta tray bake on p. 196), soup toppers to sweet treats (Chickpea blondies on p. 211), chickpeas are wonderfully versatile. They're also one of the easiest ways to bump up the fibre content in any meal with half a tin (120g drained weight) adding around 8–9 grams of fibre, plus protein and minerals to boot.

Chia seeds

If fibre had a power ranking, chia seeds would sit firmly near the top. Just one tablespoon packs around 5g of fibre – a mix of both soluble and insoluble types –

making them one of the most concentrated sources you can add to your day. Incidentally, they're also a good source of protein, with two tablespoons providing 7g.

When mixed with liquid, chia seeds form a gel thanks to their mucilage fibre, a soluble type that swells and slows digestion. That means steadier blood sugar, better satiety and happy, well-fed gut microbes. Think of this gel as a digestion stabiliser, helping everything run at an even, comfortable pace.

Chia seeds are also rich in plant omega-3 fatty acids (ALA), which help calm inflammation, and polyphenols that nourish your microbiome even further. The result is a small seed with seriously supersized benefits.

Make them into jam (see my blackberry version on p. 210), add them to bread (I use it in the No knead seed loaf on page 205) or a make deliciously creamy chia puddings (there are three to choose from on page 128) and you get a fibre-packed, microbiome-loving meal in minutes. You can also grind them (as with flaxseeds, on page 68) if you're less keen on their somewhat gloopy texture, or scatter them over salads and use in baking.

Mixing 2 tablespoons of chia seeds into a small glass of water, letting them sit for 15 minutes to swell, then downing them like a shot was a viral trend known as the 'internal shower' on social media. If you can bear the texture, go for it, but please make sure you hydrate really well as that's a rapid hit of fibre.

Ground flaxseeds (also known as linseeds)

Flaxseeds are one of the most versatile fibre-boosters around. They're rich in both soluble and insoluble fibre and offer plant-based omega-3 fats. They help regulate digestion, support hormones (they contain lignans – a unique plant compound that acts a little like oestrogen, potentially helping to support hormones, particularly around perimenopause and menopause) and can help lower cholesterol.

Add to porridge (see Soaked pearl barley porridge on p. 122), granola (see Cardamon-spiced gut-loving granola on p. 127) or just sprinkle a heaped tablespoon over salads and soups for a subtle nutty flavour and an effortless 4g fibre boost.

It's important to grind flaxseeds before using to liberate the omega-3 fatty acids that are bound up inside the seed. You can buy them ready ground, but I buy them in kilo bags as they're more cost-effective and then grind them in small batches (around 150g at a time) in a coffee or spice grinder. You can store the ground flaxseeds in an airtight container in the fridge to keep it fresh for up to a month.

Pears

Pears are proof that fibre doesn't have to be heavy to work hard. Beneath that delicate skin lies a perfect balance of soluble and insoluble fibre, making pears a gentle but effective aid for digestion. The star here is pectin, a soluble fibre that helps lower cholesterol, steady blood sugar and feed your beneficial bacteria.

Pears also bring a dose of sorbitol, a natural sugar alcohol that draws water into the bowel and helps things stay regular – ideal if your digestion tends to be on the slower side. Other good sources of sorbitol include stone-based fruits like apricots, peaches, nectarines, dates and prunes.

A medium-sized pear boasts 4g fibre. Check out the Maple pecan baked pears on p. 132 for a delicious way to eat them for breakfast.

Kiwi fruit

Don't be fooled by their size, kiwis punch well above their weight when it comes to fibre and gut health. Each one delivers around 2g fibre, plus they contain a special digestive enzyme called actinidin, which helps break down proteins and keeps things moving comfortably through your gut. Think of actinidin as a little enzymatic assistant, helping your digestive system work more efficiently, which can be especially useful after heavier meals and makes them a great dessert.

Kiwis are also rich in pectin (see Pears, above) that helps form those satisfying, easy-to-pass poos we all secretly appreciate. In fact, studies have shown that eating two kiwis a day can improve bowel regularity as effectively as fibre supplements.

And the benefits don't stop there: the combination of fibre, vitamin C and antioxidants makes kiwi a total all-rounder for immunity, skin and energy. For the full effect, keep the skin on – it's completely edible, packed with extra insoluble fibre and surprisingly pleasant once you get used to the texture. Look for golden kiwis that are slightly less hairy and have thinner skins, which makes this a little easier! I've used kiwis in the Soaked pearl barley porridge on p. 122 and they make a great snack – I eat them like apples and my kids cut them in half and scoop out the flesh with a spoon.

Berries

Berries are where flavour, fibre and science collide. Whether you're team raspberry, blueberry, blackberry or strawberry, berries are fibre-rich powerhouses, with most offering around 4–6g fibre per 100g (depending on the variety). Berries, such as raspberries and blackberries, are aggregate fruits, i.e. they are made up of lots of tiny, individual berries (known as drupelets) clustered together to form a whole berry. Each drupelet has a thin skin and contains a seed, making these types of berries particularly high in fibre.

The fibre in berries also helps slow the absorption of natural sugars, meaning they're sweet but won't elevate your blood sugar. And thanks to their high water content, they're hydrating and gentle on digestion.

Frozen berries are just as nutritious as fresh, often cheaper and are available year-round. Add them to porridge, yoghurt, smoothies or chia puddings for a colourful fibre boost that feels like a treat. You'll find frozen berries in the Raspberry and pecan black bean brownies on p. 218 – a surprising hit with my kids – and in the blackberry chia jam in the Toasted rye porridge recipe on p. 134.

Broccoli

Broccoli might not have the glamour of berries or the trend factor of chia, but it's one of the most powerful foods you can put on your plate. A cupped handful of broccoli gives you 2.5g fibre. But fibre is just the beginning. Broccoli also contains sulforaphane, a unique compound formed when it's chopped or chewed, which has powerful anti-inflammatory and antioxidant effects. Think of it as your gut's internal clean-up crew, working behind the scenes to keep you healthy.

Lightly steaming broccoli keeps that sulforaphane active, while pairing it with a drizzle of olive oil helps you absorb its fat-soluble nutrients like vitamin K. Whether it's in a stir-fry, soup or roasted traybake, broccoli is one of the simplest ways to give your gut, hormones and immune system a daily boost. There's no need to waste any of the plant, either. I've made the head into a 'rice' (see p. 172) and the stalk into 'fries' (see p. 202). And don't forget you can get a wide range of different types from Tenderstem to purple sprouting.

Peas and edamame beans

Peas and edamame might come from different plants – one a classic garden staple, the other a young soybean – but nutritionally, they come from the same pod. Both deliver a powerful mix of fibre and plant protein, making them ideal for balancing blood sugar, feeding your gut microbes and keeping you feeling full and satisfied.

We often talk about protein and fibre as if they're in competition – one for muscle, the other for digestion – but these two ingredients prove they're actually a dream team. In fact, peas and edamame beans cover both bases beautifully: around 4–6g fibre and up to 10g protein per 80g serving in the case of edamame beans. Together, they help trigger appetite-regulating hormones like PYY and GLP-1, signalling to your brain that you're full and keeping your energy and mood stable long after you've eaten.

They're also rich in polyphenols, folate and vitamin K and they support regular digestion and a diverse microbiome. Frozen versions are just as nutritious as fresh and often much cheaper.

Think of peas and edamame as your green multi-taskers: easy, affordable and the perfect bridge between the protein and fibre worlds. They cook in minutes and are the ultimate convenience ingredient: toss them into salads (see Miso salmon/tofu plant bowl on p. 190), soups (Pea and mint soup on p. 156), risottos or stir-fries, or combine them (Smashed peas and edamame beans on rye on p. 130) for a plant-powered boost that's also high in protein.

Sweet potatoes

Sweet potatoes are proof that comfort food and fibre can absolutely coexist. Beneath their vibrant orange skin lies a powerhouse of soluble and insoluble fibre, helping to keep your digestion regular, feed your gut microbes and support steady blood sugar levels.

Their natural sweetness comes with a low glycaemic load, meaning they release energy slowly. That's thanks, in part, to their pectin and resistant starch, which act as natural slow burners and prebiotics. They're also rich in beta-carotene, the antioxidant your body converts to vitamin A, supporting skin, vision and immune health. A medium-sized baked sweet potato will give you around 4.5g fibre.

Roast them, mash them, cube them into curries or even slice them and pop them in the toaster, sweet potatoes are endlessly versatile and deeply satisfying. They work beautifully in my Sweet potato with freekeh and whipped tahini on p. 160.

Beans

If there's one ingredient that deserves a standing ovation in the fibre world, it's beans. Whether you're into black, kidney, cannellini or butter beans, they're all bursting with soluble and insoluble fibre, plant protein and resistant starch – a triple whammy for gut health and balanced energy.

Some varieties are true standouts. Red kidney beans and borlotti beans top the list at around 8.5g fibre per ½ tin (120g drained weight), followed closely by haricot beans (the ones used in baked beans), black beans, cannellini and pinto beans – all hovering around 7g. Even lighter options, like butter beans, still deliver a solid 5g per ½ can, which is a huge return for something so simple to add to meals. Speaking of baked beans, they're an affordable, familiar and genuinely useful source of fibre and plant protein, especially when time or energy is low. A small 150g can gives you a very impressive 7.5g fibre. Yes, they're considered an ultra-processed food (somewhat unfairly in my opinion), but paired with wholegrain toast or added on top of a baked potato, they make a simple, comforting meal that still supports your gut (just opt for sugar-free, low-salt options where possible).

Like peas, beans perfectly blur the line between protein and fibre; no need to choose between the two. They're also rich in minerals like magnesium, iron and potassium and their slow-release nature helps you feel satisfied for hours.

Tinned beans are every busy cook's secret weapon. Toss them into soups, stews, salads and pasta dishes, or blend into dips for a creamy, fibre-packed upgrade. I've used them liberally throughout the recipes, check out Harissa mixed bean stew on p. 198, the Black bean burger on p. 178, Easy minestrone on p. 150 and Borlotti bean ragú on p. 180. I've even included them in my brownies on p. 218 and no, I swear you can't taste them!

Nuts and seeds

Nuts and seeds are the ultimate fibre snack: small, portable and packed with goodness. They deliver a marvellous mix of soluble and insoluble fibre, plant protein, healthy fats and a host of micronutrients like magnesium, zinc and vitamin E.

Almonds and pistachios weigh in at around 3.5g fibre per 30g handful, pumpkin seeds have 3g, sunflower seeds and pecans have around 2g, with cashews and walnuts not far behind at 1.5g.

The beauty of nuts and seeds is their flexibility: sprinkle them on porridge, yoghurt or salads; blend into smoothies; stir into baking; or simply enjoy a handful on their own as a snack. They're an easy, everyday way to boost fibre intake, support gut health and get a bit of protein without even thinking about it. Check out my Cardamom-spiced gut-loving granola on p. 127 and the No-knead seed loaf on p. 205.

Toasting nuts and seeds can bring out a wonderful nutty flavour and works well when adding spices or herbs and eating them as a snack. I just add them to a hot dry frying pan and cook for a few minutes, being careful to keep them moving so they turn golden but don't burn. Keep them in an airtight container and add a tablespoon to meals wherever possible.

Lentils

If there's a quiet overachiever in the fibre world, it's lentils. Just half a tin of cooked lentils (118g drained weight) delivers around 6g fibre, plus plant protein, iron and zinc. Their secret strength lies in their mix of soluble and insoluble fibre. Lentils also release energy slowly, supporting steady blood sugar levels and helping you feel satisfied for longer.

But the magic doesn't stop there. Lentils are a favourite food of your gut microbes, who ferment their fibres to produce those powerful short-chain fatty acids we talked about on page 35 – the ones that help calm inflammation, support your immune system and protect your gut lining. Think of lentils as tiny, edible fertiliser for a thriving, resilient microbiome.

They're also wonderfully affordable, gentle on the planet and incredibly adaptable. From dahls, stews and soups to salads, pasta sauces and even blended into dips, lentils are one of the easiest ways to weave more fibre into everyday meals. For a microbiome-boosting combo, try pairing them with colourful vegetables (rich in polyphenols) and wholegrains like brown rice or barley: simple, hearty, gut-loving food at its best – try my 50:50 spag bol on p. 174 and Dahl with roasted carrots and egg on p. 186 to see them in action.

Other wholegrains

Other wholegrains, like brown rice, quinoa, freekeh, bulgur, barley, rye and buckwheat are your slow-release energy champions. Aim to mix your grains up through the week. Try swapping white pasta for wholewheat, white bread for seeded and wholegrain varieties, white rice for black, red, brown or wild, and try different varieties of wholegrains like barley, rye or quinoa. I rely on pre-cooked pouches because they save so much time – many contain simply the grain and a little olive oil. It's also a great way to try new grains without buying a large bag only to find you – or your family – aren't that keen.

Pearl barley boasts 4.5g fibre per 100g (cooked) and features in the Tomato and red pepper pearl barley risotto on p. 158 and one of my favourite breakfasts, Soaked pearl barley porridge with kiwi on p. 122. Quinoa has 4g per 100g and makes up the base of lots of my nourish bowls (see Chicken, avocado and quinoa nourish bowl with herb dressing on p. 144). I've used freekeh – with 1.5g per 100g cooked weight – as the base for my Halloumi power bowl with figs and honey-lemon dressing on p. 149. Rye flakes (4.5g per 30g serving) and barley flakes (3g per 30g serving) are good alternatives to oats and can be used for porridge or in baking. Note that buckwheat (1.5g per 30g serving) and quinoa flakes (1g per 30g serving) are gluten-free and cook fairly quickly, compared to rye and barley flakes, which will take a little longer to cook than regular oats but are worth the investment when you have time.

Onions, garlic and leeks

These all belong to the allium family and are rich in the soluble fibre inulin, as well as fructans, both of which act as powerful prebiotics (see p. 37). As well as feeding our beneficial gut bacteria and supporting digestion, they even help with mineral absorption.

Regularly using alliums in cooking is one of the easiest ways to boost fibre and flavour at once, but because inulin ferments quickly in the gut, some people may find they cause bloating and gastrointestinal discomfort. In fact, all foods in the onion family can cause issues for people with IBS. If that's you, try substituting the green tops of spring onions and chives for onion when cooking, or use garlic-infused olive oil for flavour, as these tend to be better tolerated. You won't get the full health benefits of eating garlic, but flavour is just as important!

Roast whole garlic bulbs until soft and sweet and simply squeeze them out of their shells before blending into the base for soups, stews and sauces (see below). Finely sliced leeks add a delicate flavour (see the Quick ribollita on p. 170 and Leek, broccoli and potato soup on p. 152), while raw onions or crushed garlic bring a sharp, probiotic-friendly kick to dressings, dips and sauces. For example, I've included a clove of raw garlic in the burger sauce recipe on p. 178.

How to roast a whole garlic bulb

Simply cut the top off the garlic bulb, exposing the very tops of the cloves. Place the bulb on a small square of baking paper or foil, and drizzle with olive oil. Season with salt and pepper. Scrunch up the paper or foil to seal in the bulb and roast at 180°C (160°C fan)/350°F for 30–40 minutes.

When cooked, the garlic should be soft when pressed and the papery outside case will have turned a golden colour. Leave to cool for a few minutes before squeezing the soft roasted garlic out of their shells.

Leafy greens (e.g. kale, spring greens, watercress, spinach, rocket, pak choi, bok choy)

Don't underestimate your greens: they might look lightweight, but they're fibre-rich, mineral-packed (especially when it comes to iron and magnesium) and full of phytonutrients that support gut, hormone and immune health. Mixing them up gives your microbiome a variety of plant compounds to thrive on and they've been linked to better brain health, too.

Add a handful to soups, smoothies, curries or omelettes – or mix multiple greens for a fibre-packed salad base that you can build on. Opt for baby spinach if you're eating your greens raw – it has fewer oxalates, which can bind with minerals like calcium and lower your ability to absorb them – or simply lightly cook it (wilting or steaming), which will lower the oxalates, too. Kale tops the list at 3.2g per 100g, with cavolo nero not far behind at 3.1g. Check out my Cavolo nero anchovy linguine on p. 194 for a delicious way to get your greens in. Spring greens have around 3g per 100g, pak choi and rocket 1.7g and spinach and watercress 1.5g. You'll find spinach in the Veg-squeezed mac and cheese on p. 182, and kale in the Coconut lentils with crispy kale on p. 146.

Unexpected fibre co-stars

While beans, veg and wholegrains do the heavy lifting, there are also lesser-known foods that contribute meaningful amounts of fibre. Think of these as the side-kicks that can quietly help close the gap between where you are and your 30g goal.

Dark chocolate (at least 70% cocoa solids)

Dark chocolate is made from cocoa solids, which are naturally high in fibre and polyphenols. Generally, the higher the cocoa content, the more fibre you get: roughly 3g per 30g chocolate with 70% cocoa solids, and 4g for 30g made with 85% cocoa solids. This increases to a very impressive 5g of fibre per heaped tablespoon of powdered cacao, as it's more concentrated.

How to use: Choose chocolate containing at least 70% cocoa solids, and the fewer ingredients on the packet label the better. Sprinkle finely chopped chocolate or cacao nibs over porridge, mix into yoghurt or melt into baking for a rich, satisfying boost. You can also use cacao and cocoa powder in recipes such as the Raspberry and pecan black bean brownies on p. 218 and the Chocolate and hazelnut chia pudding on p. 128.

Coffee

Good news for the coffee fans: brewed coffee actually contains dietary fibre! Around 2g per cup with most of it being soluble fibre, which can help with digestion. Darker roasts and espressos tend to have slightly higher amounts.

How to use: Enjoy it brewed as usual, or add to chia puddings and overnight oats for a 'tiramisu' vibe.

Shredded coconut

Shredded coconut is made from the dried flesh of mature coconuts, giving it a naturally sweet flavour and chewy texture. It's a great source of insoluble fibre, coming in at about 5–7g per 30g serving. Unlike coconut sugar or coconut milk, shredded coconut retains its fibrous structure, making it a satisfying addition to both sweet and savoury dishes.

How to use: Sprinkle over porridge, yoghurt or fruit; stir into homemade granola or energy bites; or use as a coating for energy balls, like those on p. 213. Just be mindful that it's quite energy dense, with 1 tablespoon providing around 100 calories.

Green bananas

Most people wait until bananas are yellow to eat them, but before they ripen their starch hasn't yet converted to sugar, meaning green bananas are packed with resistant starch. You'll remember we spoke about this on page 30, which your gut microbes – particularly the butyrate-producers – love to munch on. Green bananas are less sweet and more firm than ripe bananas, offering slow-release energy and excellent prebiotic benefits.

How to use: Blend into smoothies (they thicken them beautifully), mash them and add to muffins or porridge for a subtle, sweet flavour, or slice and pair with nut butter on toast. Try using them in the Chickpea blondies on p. 211 and the Soaked pearl barley porridge on p. 122.

Popcorn

Popcorn is a wholegrain that's often overlooked as a fibre food. When popped, it provides around 4.5g of fibre per 30g serving, making it a satisfying (and low-calorie at 110 cals) snack option. Its insoluble fibre supports regular digestion, while its crunch makes it a good alternative to crisps.

How to use: Air-pop and then season with cinnamon, garlic powder, smoked paprika or nutritional yeast. I'll show you how on p. 214. Or opt for a shop-bought pack, which provides 2.5g fibre per small 30g pack.

Artichokes

Globe artichokes are one of the richest vegetable sources of fibre – up to 10g per medium globe. There's a reason they're fondly known as 'fartichokes', as they're especially high in inulin (see more on this on p. 38), which can cause a lot of wind and bloating in some people. However, their earthy flavour and creamy texture make them both delicious and nutritious.

How to use: Steam or roast whole artichokes and peel away the leaves to enjoy with a drizzle of olive oil or lemon. You can also use canned or jarred artichoke hearts in salads, pasta or dips for convenience. Check out how I use them in the Miso beans on p. 154.

Basil seeds

Basil seeds (sometimes called sabja or tukmaria seeds) come from the sweet basil plant and are gaining popularity as a gentle, natural source of soluble fibre. They look and behave very much like chia seeds, swelling into a soft, jelly-like texture when soaked in liquid. In fact, basil seeds form a slightly thicker gel than chia seeds, which may make them feel even more filling. I buy mine online and like to use them interchangeably with chia seeds for variety and no, they don't taste like basil!

How to use: Use them instead of chia seeds as the base for chia puddings (see p. 128), add them to granola or sprinkle them on overnight oats or soups for a fibre boost. You can also grind them (just like flaxseeds) if you're averse to their somewhat gloopy texture. I use 1–2 tablespoons, which provides 7.5 to 15g of fibre – slightly higher than chia seeds.

Mushrooms

Mushrooms are a surprising source of fibre – around 2g per 100g – particularly the type of fibre called beta-glucans, which you'll remember is helpful for lowering cholesterol. Different varieties of mushrooms, such as shiitake, maitake and oyster mushrooms, contain slightly different blends of fibres and plant compounds, all of which feed beneficial gut bacteria. Dried mushrooms are especially rich in fibre and add a deep, savoury flavour to dishes.

How to use: I learned this top tip from a renowned chef: to get the best from your mushrooms – and intensify their flavour – dry-fry them in a hot pan for 8–10 minutes, until they release their juices and start to turn golden brown. Only then do you add your oil and any flavourings, such as garlic, spices and herbs. Stir the end result into omelettes or pasta, or add dried mushrooms to soups, stews or risottos for a rich, earthy flavour. You'll find mushrooms in the base mix for the Borlotti ragú on p. 180.

Nutritional yeast

Nutritional yeast (sometimes called 'nooch') is a deactivated yeast with a naturally savoury, cheesy flavour that makes it an easy fibre-friendly addition to everyday meals. A tablespoon provides 3g fibre, along with B-vitamins (including B12 in fortified versions) and protein.

How to use: It dissolves quickly into soups, pasta, stews and salad dressings, adding depth without altering the overall dish. Think of it as an undercover enhancer – a simple sprinkle that lifts flavour while quietly nudging up your nutrient intake. I've included it in the One-pot creamy white beans on p. 162 and Easy minestrone soup on p. 150.

Do I need a fibre supplement?

Ideally, all of your fibre should come from food. Wholegrains, fruit, vegetables, pulses, nuts and seeds don't just provide fibre, but a host of vitamins, minerals and plant compounds, too. That said, getting enough every day isn't always easy. Travel and holidays can throw routines off – meals out, different time zones and less access to your usual foods can all make fibre harder to come by. Illness can change your appetite or make you rely more on plain, lower-fibre foods. And at certain times of the month, if you have periods, digestion naturally shifts with hormonal changes, and some people find they benefit from a little extra fibre to stay regular and feel comfortable. In short: life happens, and it's normal to have days or phases where your fibre intake dips. This is where fibre supplements can play a useful, supporting role, helping to bridge the gap.

Psyllium is a soluble fibre superstar. When mixed with water, it forms a viscous gel that helps regulate digestion and supports healthy bowel movements. It's non-fermentable (i.e., it's not a prebiotic) so doesn't feed your gut bacteria, but it is brilliant for keeping things regular and has been shown to lower LDL cholesterol and steady blood sugar, too. Brands such as Metamucil use psyllium husk as the main ingredient in their fibre drinks. I've included it here in the supplement section, but it's actually a kitchen cupboard ingredient I use frequently in baking, granola and sometimes just to add some extra fibre oomph to my breakfasts.

Personally, I don't like stirring psyllium into wet ingredients (such as yoghurt or smoothies) as, in my opinion, it just isn't an enjoyable texture. It's much more appealing sprinkled on top of things, like overnight oats, just before eating. And a little goes a long way. Just 1 teaspoon gives you 5.5g fibre – that's one-sixth of your total recommended target. Always drink plenty of water alongside it, to make sure it moves freely through your gut. I've used psyllium in the No-knead seed loaf on p. 205, the Pear and courgette cake on p. 216 and the Cardamon-spiced granola on p. 127.

Inulin is a natural prebiotic fibre derived from chicory root but it can be tricky for some people. It ferments quite quickly in the gut – mainly in the early part of the colon – which can lead to bloating and excess gas soon after eating. If you have IBS (which means you're often more sensitive to high FODMAP foods such as garlic, onions and leeks), you may notice these effects more strongly, in which case inulin powder is probably not best for you and you may want to avoid it.

Partially hydrolysed guar gum (PHGG) is a gentle soluble fibre made from guar beans that has a bowel-normalising effect – i.e. it helps with both diarrhoea and constipation. It's well tolerated (even for people with IBS) and mixes easily into drinks without thickening or affecting taste. Research suggests it supports beneficial gut bacteria and can help ease both constipation and diarrhoea.

Custom prebiotic fibre blends (Myota, LOAM and similar brands) are blends of different prebiotic fibres that can support gut health and encourage microbial diversity. They typically offer around 10g fibre per serving and combine a number of different prebiotic fibres, including hydrolysed guar gum, acacia fibre, tapioca, wheat dextrin, cellulose and other soluble fibres designed to nourish a range of beneficial bacteria. You add the powder to water (or coffee, shakes or smoothies) once daily, but because custom blends often contain fermentable ingredients, start slowly to gauge tolerance.

Konjac (glucomannan) is a root vegetable that grows in Asia. It's ground and sometimes sold as a supplement or is often made into noodles (sometimes called shirataki or 'skinny' noodles). Konjac absorbs liquids and so needs to be consumed with plenty of water. Not advised for anyone who has IBS.

A note on choosing fibre supplements wisely

Not all fibre supplements are equal. Look for products with clear labelling, simple ingredient lists and no added sugars or artificial sweeteners if possible. Start with small amounts and increase gradually to allow your gut to adapt. If in doubt, leave it out and focus on foods instead, they're hands down the best option.

Probiotic supplements

We've already discussed on p. 39 how probiotics in food – e.g. kimchi, kefir, yoghurt, miso and sauerkraut – can benefit health, but what about live bacteria from supplements? Research shows that certain probiotic strains in supplement form can help with issues like antibiotic-associated diarrhoea, irritable bowel syndrome (IBS), constipation and some immune responses. But probiotic supplements aren't a one-size-fits-all solution: their effects are strain-specific, meaning different strains do different jobs, and not every product will work for every person or every condition.

It's also important to know that taking probiotic supplements doesn't permanently 'reseed' your gut. For most people, they act more like temporary visitors – supporting the existing community, nudging your microbiome in a helpful direction and influencing gut signalling, immune function and barrier health while they are present. Once you stop taking them, their benefits may fade, which is why they tend to work best as part of a broader gut-supportive lifestyle rather than a standalone fix.

There's promising research in areas like mood, immunity and metabolic health, but the science is still evolving and not all supplements on the market have clinical backing. If you want to try one, look for a product that specifies the strain(s) and has research behind it, and give it at least 8–12 weeks to see how you respond. And remember: for most of us, eating a diverse, fibre-rich diet is still the most powerful and reliable way to support a thriving microbiome – probiotic supplements can possibly be a useful extra layer, but they are certainly not a replacement.

Probiotic strains and their uses

- ***Lactobacillus rhamnosus*:** Helpful during and after antibiotic treatment to reduce diarrhoea and traveller's tummy.
- ***Bifodobacterium lactis*:** Supports the immune system, especially in the case of upper respiratory infections.
- ***Lactobacillus acidophilus*:** Helps support the vaginal microbiome to reduce bacterial vaginosis and thrush.
- ***Saccharomyces boulardii*:** A yeast often used during or after antibiotic use to repopulate the gut microbiome.

Now you have a clearer understanding of the key fibre sources, the next step is making fibre fit easily into your life. In Chapter 3, we'll look at smart shopping choices, tips for maximising fibre and a 10-day challenge to kick-start this new habit – plus how to deal with common side effects of upping your fibre.

Your fibre-friendly life

Now that you understand the magic of fibre and the science behind why it matters, it's time to bring it off the page and into your everyday life. This chapter is your practical playbook: the simple food swaps, shopping strategies and clever cooking hacks that make eating more fibre feel natural, joyful and totally doable – even on busy days. You'll learn how to stock your kitchen without spending a fortune, how to build meals that keep your gut happy and energy steady and how to increase fibre gradually (and comfortably) with smart tweaks. From a 10-day challenge to a gentle guide to embracing beans, consider this your step-by-step blueprint for turning fibre into a habit, not a hassle.

Shop clever

One of the easiest ways to eat more fibre isn't about complicated recipes or fancy superfoods, it's about what you keep stocked and ready to go – this is how I've built most of the recipes in this book. When your cupboards are filled with simple, nourishing staples, it makes it so much easier to reach your fibre goals.

These are the smart buys that make it easy to throw together a meal that keeps you feeling full and your gut happy. A spoonful here, a sprinkle there – it all adds up. Think of this list as your baseline fibre toolkit: reliable, versatile and packed with ingredients that multitask across breakfast, lunch and dinner.

Bread

Not all bread is created equal. Look for seeded loaves, rye bread, sprouted seed bread such as Ezekiel and pumpernickel, or sourdough with wholegrains. Be aware that just because something is labelled as wholemeal, it doesn't make it high fibre. Check the numbers: 6g fibre per 100g (or more) puts bread in high-fibre territory. If you want an easy DIY option, try my No-knead seed loaf on p. 205, which has 10g fibre per slice and tastes next level. Bread is such an easy way to put together a meal and boost fibre – served as a side with soups, such as Easy minestrone on p. 150, or as the base of Miso beans and artichoke hearts on pesto toast on p. 154 – so it's worth choosing wisely.

Cereals

Breakfast cereals can be secret fibre heroes or sneaky sugar bombs with health halos. The key is to look beyond the front-of-pack promises. Aim for at least 6g fibre per 100g and you want any added sugars to be low on the ingredients list. Options with whole oats, wheat bran or barley are usually your best bet. Think bran flakes, Weetabix-style biscuits and oat-based blends. Avoid cereals where the first ingredient is sugar (yes, even the ones claiming to be wholegrain).

Tip: If your existing cereal isn't super high in fibre, don't ditch it, boost it. Stir in chia or flaxseeds, sprinkle on nuts, and top with berries to fibre-boost in seconds.

Cereal cheat sheet

Top-tier fibre heroes
- All-Bran/wheat bran cereals: usually the highest-fibre options in the aisle (11g fibre per 40g serving).
- Bran flakes (7g per 40g serving).
- Shredded wheat/bite-size shredded wheat: simple, wholegrain, no fuss (6.5g fibre per 2 biscuit servings).
- Weetabix and supermarket wheat biscuits: reliable breakfast staple (4g per 2-biscuit serving).
- Porridge oats/oat bran/jumbo oats: classic slow-release fibre favourite (3.5–5g fibre per 40g serving).

Solid everyday choices
- No-added-sugar muesli (look for oats, barley or wheat mixes rather than mostly dried fruit).
- Oat-based granolas – choose low-sugar versions; some are fibre-rich but sugar-heavy.

Try my Cardamom-spiced gut-loving granola on p. 127 for a low-sugar, high-fibre (4.5g per 40g) alternative.

Tip: Boost lower-fibre options with a tablespoon of ground flaxseeds or a sprinkle of nuts, or add a cupped handful of berries to easily add an extra 5–8g fibre.

Cautions
*   'Wholegrain' on the box doesn't automatically mean high fibre: check for ≥6g per 100g.
*   Added fibre claims (e.g. chicory root/inulin) can help, but shouldn't be your only fibre source.
*   Granolas can be sneaky sugar traps: aim for <5g sugar/100g when possible.

Dark rye crackers/crispbreads

Rye crispbreads (like Ryvita) and oatcakes are simple and genuinely useful cupboard staples – long shelf life, instant crunch, big fibre bump. Depending on the brand, you'll get about 1.5–1.9g fibre per slice. Use instead of toast with eggs, hummus, avocado or cottage cheese for a retro classic! You could also crumble them on top of soups such as Quick ribollita on p. 170 or Easy minestrone soup on p. 150, in place of bread croutons.

Tinned goods

Don't overlook the tins aisle: it's a fibre goldmine. Tinned beans, lentils and chickpeas are budget-friendly, pre-cooked and ready to throw into salads, soups and curries. They are the basis of so many of the recipes in this book, including: Black bean and herb avocado toast on p. 124, Crushed chickpea-stuffed pitta on p. 143, Black bean burger on p. 178 and Chickpea blondies on p. 211. Just rinse before using to remove excess fermentable compounds if you're easing into fibre. Keep a few tins in your cupboard and you'll always have an instant fibre boost on hand.

Frozen berries

Frozen berries are a brilliant, budget-friendly staple. They're picked at peak ripeness (so just as nutritious as fresh), packed with fibre and antioxidants, and perfect for porridge, yoghurt bowls and smoothies. Plus, they won't go mushy in the fruit bowl – fewer sad berries in the bin, more fibre in your bowl. I've used frozen cherries in the Cherry bakewell overnight oats on p. 125 and I've used frozen blackberries in the Blackberry chia jam on p. 210.

Frozen veg

Frozen spinach, onions, peas, cauliflower, broccoli, sweetcorn, edamame beans and mixed veg keep for ages and are fibre heroes in disguise. They go straight from the freezer to the pan and lock in their nutrients. Add to soups, curries, pasta sauces and smoothies. Check out the Smashed peas and edamame beans on rye on p. 130 and my Leek, broccoli and potato soup on p. 152, which both work well with frozen veg. I also swear by frozen 'soffrito' as the base for my Quick ribolitta on p. 170 and One-pot creamy white beans on p. 162, rather than chopping carrots, celery and onions – it saves so much time!

Mixed packs of fruit and veg

Buy variety in one go by choosing mixed packs, like a trio of peppers, a medley of tomatoes or a bag of mixed leafy greens. Each colour brings a slightly different type of fibre and plant compound, so these packs make it easy to tick off diversity plant points without overthinking it. Think of them as ready-made microbiome boosters.

Pre-chopped and pre-cooked lifesavers

Bagged salads, chopped stir-fry mixes, brown rice, freekeh, quinoa or lentil pouches – these aren't cheats, they're fibre facilitators. If convenience gets you eating more plants, it counts. One of my absolute go-to meals that I make every week is the Greens and beans taco salad on p. 188, which uses a pack of mixed leafy greens alongside some black beans and herbs and is on the table in less than 20 minutes.

Plant-protein champions

Tofu, tempeh, edamame beans, tinned lentils, mixed beans, chia seeds and peas bring fibre *and* protein to your meals, helping to keep you full and feeding your gut microbes. They're double-duty ingredients worth making space for in your fridge and cupboard.

Pasta

No need to forgo pasta, you just have to pick the right one. Wholewheat pasta is usually the simplest swap, offering 6–8g fibre per 100g compared to around 2–3g in white pasta. If you want to push things further, look for legume-based varieties (red lentil, chickpea, pea, mung bean): they come in at around 10–15g fibre per 100g and boast extra protein to keep you satisfied. Texture-wise, wholewheat pasta has a lovely nutty bite, and legume pastas hold sauce brilliantly. And don't worry if you (or your family) love your traditional pasta, no need to ditch it – just mix half and half. I've used mung bean pasta in the Cavolo nero anchovy linguine recipe on p. 194, which ramps the fibre up to a whopping 21g per serving.

Noodles

Noodles don't have to be off the table, either, just choose ones that give you a fibre boost. Wholewheat or buckwheat soba noodles are great everyday options, usually offering 3–5g of fibre per 100g compared to the 1–2g in many white rice noodles. If you enjoy Asian-style meals, also look out for edamame or mung bean noodles, which can climb to 8–12g fibre per 100g and pack in extra protein, too. Texture-wise, wholewheat noodles have a slightly chewier bite and work beautifully in stir-fries, broths and noodle bowls. And as with pasta, if your family prefers the classic kind, simply mix them together – a little upgrade can go a long way. I used buckwheat noodles in the Crispy chilli oil buckwheat noodles on p. 148, which taste great and offer plenty of fibre.

Wraps

To maximise fibre, look for wholegrain options and aim for at least 5–6g of fibre per wrap (many white wraps sit at just 1–2g). Wholemeal tortillas, seeded flatbreads and oat-based wraps tend to perform best, and they often keep you fuller for longer thanks to their slower-release carbs and extra nutrients. Wraps often fall into the ultra-processed category, so check out Crosta & Mollica, which only have four ingredients – flour, water, extra virgin olive oil and salt – or make the Red lentil wraps on p. 206, which I use for speedy lunches when I'm working from home. They work well with sweet or savoury fillings, are vegan, gluten-free and keep in the fridge for up to 3 days. I also like filling them with leftover Raw pad Thai on p. 166 for a fuss-free, filling portable lunch.

Snacks

Don't be fooled by things like lentil crisps or rice cakes, they often have around the same amount – or even less – fibre than regular crisps. If you're a crisp fan (I am!), you might want to look at including baked crisps over regular ones – it's not a huge difference at 1.6g compared to 1g – but every little helps. If you want high-fibre snack options, check out my Crispy garlic beans on p. 204 and the two popcorn options on p. 214 or, if in doubt, always carry some mixed nuts with you. Be sure to check out my Chickpea blondies on p. 211, Cookie dough energy balls on p. 213 and Healthier oat bran cookies on p. 212, too, if you want something sweet but filling.

From low to high: Everyday fibre fixes

Small swaps can offer big gains. Here are some examples of how to level up your fibre intake in everyday meals, without giving up flavour.

Breakfast

Before: White toast with butter and jam ($\approx$ 1g)
After: Wholegrain toast with peanut butter and sliced banana ($\approx$ 6g)
→ *Adds +5g fibre*

Before: Cornflakes with milk ($\approx$ 1g)
After: Overnight oats topped with berries, chia seeds and honey ($\approx$ 10g)
→ *Adds +9g fibre*

Before: Plain yoghurt with honey ($\approx$ 0g)
After: Greek yoghurt parfait with oats, flaxseed and diced pear ($\approx$ 7g)
→ *Adds +7g fibre*

Before: White bagel with cream cheese ($\approx$ 2g)
After: Wholegrain bagel with avocado and tomato slices ($\approx$ 8g)
→ *Adds +6g fibre*

Lunch

Before: White rice with stir-fried chicken ($\approx$ 1g)
After: Brown rice or quinoa bowl with chicken, veggies and edamame ($\approx$ 8g)
→ *Adds +7g fibre*

Before: White wrap with ham and cheese ($\approx$ 1g)
After: Wholegrain wrap with hummus, spinach, peppers and grilled tofu or chicken ($\approx$ 9g)
→ *Adds +8g fibre*

Before: Instant noodles ($\approx$ 2g)
After: Buckwheat soba noodles or lentil pasta with mixed greens, tofu and sesame dressing ($\approx$ 10g)
→ *Adds +8g fibre*

Before: Caesar salad with croutons ($\approx$ 2g)
After: Mixed bean salad with chickpeas, kale and roasted sweet potato ($\approx$ 11g)
→ *Adds +9g fibre*

Dinner

Before: White pasta with cream sauce ($\approx$ 2g)
After: Lentil or wholewheat pasta with tomato and veg sauce and seeds ($\approx$ 12g)
→ *Adds +10g fibre*

Before: Ready-made (shop-bought) white mashed potato and steak ($\approx$ 3g)
After: Mashed sweet potato (skin on) and steak ($\approx$ 11g)
→ *Adds +8g fibre*

Before: Chicken korma with pilau rice and naan ($\approx$ 4g)
After: Chana masala (chickpea curry) with brown basmati rice and wholemeal roti ($\approx$ 14g)
➔ *Adds +10g fibre*

Before: Classic white rice mushroom risotto ($\approx$ 2g)
After: Pearl barley risotto with mushrooms, peas and spinach ($\approx$ 10g)
➔ *Adds +8g fibre*

Snack

Before: Packet of crisps ($\approx$ 1g)
After: Packet of popcorn ($\approx$ 3g)
➔ *Adds +2g fibre*

Before: 50g of milk chocolate ($\approx$ 1g)
After: 50g of 85% dark chocolate ($\approx$ 6.5g)
➔ *Adds +5.5g fibre*

Before: White bread sandwich with ham and cheese ($\approx$ 1g)
After: Wholemeal pitta pocket with hummus and salad ($\approx$ 6g)
➔ *Adds +5g fibre*

Before: Handful pretzels ($\approx$ 1g)
After: Handful mixed nuts ($\approx$ 3g)
➔ *Adds +2g fibre*

The 10-day fibre challenge

If you're not quite ready to leap to 30g of fibre a day, consider this your stepping stone. It's a zero-fuss challenge to help you add a bit more fibre to your life – day by day. One of the most important daily habits when you're upping fibre is to drink around 2 litres of water, so make that a non-negotiable from the outset.

Day 1: Eat 2 kiwi fruit	Great for digestion and regularity. Some studies suggest they also help with sleep (bonus!). **Pro tip:** Eat them with the skin on (yes really!) for extra fibre.
Day 2: Add 1 tbsp ground flaxseed to a meal	Stir into porridge, yoghurt or sprinkle over a salad. **Pro tip:** Keep ground flaxseeds in the fridge to preserve those healthy fats.
Day 3: Eat a rainbow plate	Aim for 3 different-coloured veg at dinner. **Pro tip:** Try a diversity bowl, such as the Warm winter nourish bowl on p. 164.
Day 4: Eat a cupped handful of cruciferous veg	Broccoli, cauliflower, cabbage or Brussels sprouts. **Pro tip:** Try the Roasted Brussels sprouts with Parmesan on p. 203 – the cheese is a game-changer for persuading kids!
Day 5: Add a tablespoon of psyllium husk on top of yoghurt or overnight oats	Very effective for gut regularity. **Pro tip:** Start with 1 teaspoon if you're new to it and build up.

Day 6: Add a tablespoon of mixed seeds to a meal	Pumpkin, sunflower, sesame, hemp, poppy, chia, flax … add fibre *and* plant points effortlessly. **Pro tip:** Keep a diversity jar that combines lots of them on your dining table as a reminder to sprinkle over everything.
Day 7: Try a legume-based pasta	Chickpea or lentil pasta = fibre + protein. **Pro tip:** Mix half-and-half with regular pasta if you're new to them (see my 50:50 spag bol on p. 174 for inspo).
Day 8: Add a handful of berries to breakfast	Raspberries, blackberries, blueberries – all brilliant. **Pro tip:** Frozen berries are just as nutritious (and budget-friendly).
Day 9: Add some beans or lentils to lunch	Toss into soups, wraps or salads. **Pro tip:** Try the Crushed chickpea-stuffed pitta on p. 143 for a super easy but filling idea.
Day 10: Use nutritional yeast in place of Parmesan	Great on pasta, in sauces, on popcorn (see p. 215) or stirred into risottos and soups – anywhere you want a cheesy-tasting hit. **Pro tip:** Sprinkle over Easy minestrone soup (p. 150), Quick ribolitta (p. 170) or Leek, broccoli and potato soup (p. 152) or stir into the bechamel sauce in the Veg-squeezed mac and cheese on p. 182.

Now you've had 10 days of gently increasing your fibre, you may be ready to try the recipes in the next part of the book. Or, if that feels too much, continue with the challenge until you feel primed to make the leap. Alternatively, take a look at the fibre-stacking ideas on p. 102 for ways to add an extra 5g of fibre each day.

Fibre stacking:
30 easy ways to get 5g

Sometimes, the easiest way to reach 30g of fibre a day isn't by overhauling your entire diet, but by making a few small, strategic upgrades. That's where *fibre stacking* comes in. Think of it as adding quick, effortless 'boosters' to the meals you're already eating – a spoonful here, a handful there – each one delivering roughly 5g fibre. These simple additions can transform an ordinary meal into a fibre-rich one without too much extra planning or fuss. If 30g a day currently feels out of reach, fibre stacking is your gentle, achievable stepping stone.

Food	Measurement to get 5g of fibre
Fruit	
Mixed berries	140g
Oranges	2 large fruits
Pear	1 large fruit
Raspberries	30 berries
Coconut	2 tbsp
Prunes	8 dried
Vegetables	
Peas	80g
Green beans	120g
Broccoli	150g
Carrots	2 medium-sized
Sweet potato	1 medium-sized
Avocado	1 medium
Kiwi	2.5 fruits

Legumes	
Chickpeas	2 heaped tbsp
Butter beans	80g
Lentils	75g
Edamame beans	75g
Nuts and Seeds	
Chia	1 tbsp
Flaxseeds	1 tbsp
Almonds	40g
Popcorn	35g, air-popped
Psyllium husks	1 heaped tbsp
Grains	
Quinoa	125g, cooked
Oat bran	40g
Freekeh	100g, cooked
Other	
Raw cacao	1 tbsp
85% dark chocolate	40g
Dark rye sourdough	1 slice
Dark rye Ryvita	3 crackers
Hummus	2 heaped tbsp
Nutritional yeast	25g
Mung bean pasta	60g
Tofu	150g, cooked

Beat the bloat

So, you now have a list of lovely fibre-fuelled ingredients to add to your shopping list. But let's be honest, increasing fibre can sometimes come with a few side effects. Gas, bloating and even a little cramping can be common when your digestive system is adjusting. This happens because when gut microbes are busy fermenting fibre, they produce by-products like hydrogen, methane and carbon dioxide in the process.

It's important not to pathologise normal bloating. A bit of fullness or gentle distension after a meal is completely normal. Your gut is simply doing its job. That said, persistent or severe bloating, especially if accompanied by pain, unexplained weight loss, mucus or other digestive symptoms should always be checked by a GP to rule out underlying issues.

The good news is that most fibre-related bloating is temporary and usually a sign that your microbiome is waking up and doing what it's supposed to, not that something is wrong. With a few smart strategies, you can ease these symptoms and let your gut adapt comfortably, turning fibre from tummy troubler to daily superpower.

Tips I use in my clinic to manage fibre-related bloating:

- Increase fibre gradually: add an extra 5g per week on to your existing diet rather than hitting your target all at once (refer back to my fibre-stacking guide on p. 102 for quick ways to do this easily).
- Stay hydrated: fibre works best alongside water: aim for around 2 litres per day.
- Cook or steam tougher vegetables: softening fibrous foods such as broccoli makes them easier to digest. That's why I have a stir-fried broccoli rice on p. 172.
- Rinse beans and legumes: this reduces fermentable carbohydrates that can cause extra gas.

- Use a pressure cooker for beans: pressure cooking softens beans more thoroughly than standard boiling, making them easier on your gut.
- Eat slowly and chew well: smaller food particles are easier for your gut to process and reduce swallowed air which can cause bloating and gas.
- Move your body: 10–20-minute 'fart walks' after meals can help gas pass and keep digestion smooth.
- Avoid tight clothing: yoga pants, high-waisted jeans or belts that compress the stomach can worsen bloating and discomfort.
- Maintain regular mealtimes: consistent eating patterns help your digestive system run more smoothly.
- Peppermint oil capsules, fennel or mint tea: these natural remedies can relax the gut and ease bloating.
- Avoid fizzy drinks: the bubbles can increase gas and discomfort.
- Be cautious with inulin-containing foods: foods like chicory root, leeks, onions and asparagus are highly fermentable and can cause extra gas if added too quickly. Inulin may also be included in 'high-fibre' processed foods, such as protein bars and even some fizzy 'high-fibre' drinks – check labels to be sure.
- Listen to your gut: everyone's tolerance is different. Keep a food diary, note down which foods cause more bloating and adjust portions rather than eliminating them entirely.

- Front-loading your day – i.e. consuming the majority of your fibre in the daytime when your gut motility, digestive juices and colonic activity are at their strongest – may well help with bloating. Do this instead of fibre dumping, which is cramming it all into the end of the day when digestion naturally slows down a little.

If you continue to struggle with certain foods and bloating, even after putting these strategies in place, it may be worth talking to a qualified healthcare provider who can help guide you further.

Bean me up

As we've already discussed, beans are one of the best sources of fibre (and, incidentally, contain plant-based protein, too), but if you added them in as part of the 10-day challenge and perhaps felt a little bloated, or you've ever added a big serving too quickly, you'll know that it can cause a gut ruckus.

Why? Because beans contain a type of carbohydrate called oligosaccharides, which your gut microbes ferment, producing beneficial short-chain fatty acids (great!) *and* gas (not so great!). The trick is to train your gut microbes slowly, letting your system adapt week by week.

Here's your step-by-step four-week bean bootcamp training plan for those who really struggle with bloating and discomfort (feel free to swap for lentils, broccoli or whatever ingredient triggers your symptoms).

Week 1: Microdose magic
(1 teaspoon a day)

Goal: Introduce your gut to beans very gently, help it adapt.

Focus: 1 teaspoon ($\approx$ 15g) beans or lentils daily.

Tips:
- Start with the easiest-to-digest types: red lentils, split peas or mung beans.
- Add 1 teaspoon to soups, stews, to my Shakshuka with zhoug on p. 138 or blended into dips (you won't even notice them).
- Rinse tinned beans thoroughly to wash away some of the fermentable sugars.
- Drink an extra glass of water each day: hydration helps fibre move smoothly.
- Optional: add a pinch of ground cumin, ginger or fennel seeds when cooking. These traditional digestion helpers can make a difference.

Week 2: The spoonful strategy
(1–2 tablespoons a day)

Goal: Let your microbes get to know beans a little better.

Focus: Increase to 1–2 tablespoons (≈ 25–50g) beans or lentils daily.

Tips:
- Add to salads, soups (e.g. my Pea and mint soup on p. 156) or blend into hummus.
- Try lentil or mung bean pasta or soups made with red or green lentils. Try the Beef and beetroot koftas on p. 176.
- If you notice bloating, reduce portion size slightly and spread it across two meals.
- Keep up the daily water intake and try a gentle post-meal walk.
- Pressure-cook dried beans if you can, as this helps break down the gas-forming compounds.

Week 3: Confident consistency
(¼ tin or 80-100g)

Goal: Make beans a visible part of your meal.

Focus: ¼ tin ($\approx$ 60g) beans or lentils daily – can be spread across meals.

Tips:
- Add to tacos (or see the Greens and beans taco salad on p. 188), nourish bowls or pasta sauces.
- Mix beans with grains like quinoa or rice to make them easier on digestion.
- Keep a bean dip in the fridge for easy snacks.
- Introduce variety: kidney beans, chickpeas, black beans (check out Black bean and herb avocado toast on p. 124).
- Continue your fart walks (your microbes love the movement).

> # Week 4: The full portion
> ## (½ tin or 120–150g)
>
> **Goal:** Reach your fibre-friendly target with ease.
>
> **Focus:** ½ tin (≈ 120g) beans or lentils daily – can be spread across meals.
>
> **Tips:**
> - Try a bean-based stew, such as my Harissa mixed bean stew on p. 198, a curry or chilli.
> - Add beans to breakfast – try Smashed peas and edamame beans on rye on p. 130.
> - Mix different types: variety supports microbial diversity.
> - Keep an eye on hydration and mealtime regularity.
> - If bloating returns, scale back slightly and build up again – consistency wins.

Pro tips for success

Avoid dried beans until you've built up resilience. Tinned beans are better tolerated because the canning process breaks down some of the compounds (oligosaccharides) that can cause bloating. Rinsing them very, very well removes even more of these compounds and can really help with digestion.

Try adding a strip of kombu (a type of seaweed) to the cooking water – it's said to contain enzymes that help pre-digest the oligosaccharides, so they do not cause discomfort in your intestines. And while it's not exactly scientific, some spices and herbs, such as ginger, cumin and fennel, are used traditionally in some cultures to aid digestion. So these might be worth adding to your recipes, especially when cooking something like a bean stew or chickpea curry.

I've said it before but it's worth repeating here: stay well hydrated and keep moving. Fibre works best when everything's flowing.

Ultimately, if you find a food just doesn't work for you, it's not the end of the world. Fibre is so ubiquitous that, happily, you don't have to rely on one or two sources – there are literally hundreds to choose from!

Quick wins:
14 hacks to maximise fibre

Before we dive into the recipes, I want to share the simple habits that quietly underpin everything I make. These are the quick, everyday tweaks I use to naturally boost fibre without extra effort; the small things that, over time, make a big difference. You'll spot these techniques woven throughout the recipes in the next section, because this is genuinely how I cook: easy upgrades, clever shortcuts and tiny wins that slot seamlessly into real life. Think of this list as your fibre-friendly toolkit, the foundations that will help you build meals that are fuller, tastier and naturally richer in fibre.

- **Eat your skins:** Keep the skin on fruits and vegetables like potatoes, sweet potatoes, carrots, kiwis, apples, aubergines, figs and cucumbers as they contain up to 50% of the total fibre and also have many beneficial nutrients and polyphenols. I've suggested this with the kiwis in the Soaked pearl barley porridge on p. 122 and the sweet potatoes in the Sweet potato with freekeh and whipped tahini on p. 160 – just give them a good scrub first.

- **Cook smart:** Fibre isn't destroyed by heat; it stays in your food even after cooking. However, boiling can deplete levels of nutrients like vitamin C, so it's a good idea to steam or stir-fry veg when possible, to preserve the good stuff.

- **Healthy fats:** Adding a little oil such as olive oil to vegetables can help you absorb the fat-soluble vitamins they contain, such as A, D, E and K. It also adds flavour and can make vegetables much more appealing.

- **Don't rush rice:** Brown rice has its fibre-rich outer layer intact so it takes much longer than white rice to cook. Allow up to 40–50 minutes or choose pre-cooked pouches to save time.

- **Toast them:** Seeds and grains toasted in a hot dry pan before cooking can really amp up the flavour. See my Rye porridge on p. 134 as an example.

- **Mini wins:** Dried spices can contain up to 1.5g fibre per teaspoon, so add them generously to recipes to effortlessly – and deliciously – bump up the fibre *and* the polyphenol content. Cinnamon tops the list in terms of fibre (which is why I use it in so many breakfast recipes, including the chia puddings on p. 128 and the Soaked pearl barley porridge on p. 122), but garam masala, turmeric, ground coriander, cloves, curry powder, etc. are all worth having in your spice rack. You'll find them used generously throughout recipes such as Turmeric kedgeree on p. 131, Coconut lentils with crispy kale on p. 146 and Dahl with roasted carrots and egg on p. 186.

- **Fermented foods:** Not always massive fibre-hitters but great in terms of bolstering your microbiome and gut health. Try sauerkraut in your nourish bowls (see the Chicken, avocado and quinoa nourish bowl on p. 144), miso with your beans (try my Miso beans and artichoke hearts on p. 154) and kefir in your overnight oats (see p. 125).

- **Date night:** I always have some dates in my fridge to satisfy sweet cravings. I like the Medjool type, as they're softer, chewier and almost caramel-like. Sadly, they're a bit more expensive, too. One date has just over 1.5g of fibre. Slice it open and stuff with a tablespoon of crunchy peanut butter and you have a 2.5g fibre-friendly treat. I also really like them blended with nuts and seeds and rolled into balls to make a good on-the-go snack that the whole family will love – check out my Cookie dough energy bombs on p. 213.

- **Get equipped:** The right kitchen gadgets can shave lots of prep time off your meals. A simple julienne peeler is a fast and effective way to cut veg into thin strips and batons. Veg choppers make light work of dicing ingredients like onions, carrots and courgettes. And a mini-food processor is great for slicing and shredding.

- **Gluten-free:** If you're coeliac or gluten intolerant, you can still do grains. Look for buckwheat flakes, quinoa flakes, amaranth, teff and millet – feel free to swap these into any of the porridge recipes from the book. Oats are actually gluten-free but tend to be processed in factories that also handle gluten containing grains, so they can easily get cross-contaminated. Look for brands that specifically say 'gluten-free' on the packet to be sure.

- **Bread hack:** Slice and freeze your bread to avoid waste, remembering that when you toast it (from frozen) you're increasing the resistant starch (see p. 30). I always slice and freeze my No-knead seed loaf (p. 205) to make sure it lasts – it's great toasted with avocado and a crispy fried egg for a quick lunch option.

- **Amp up oats:** If you want to get maximum fibre from your oats, opt for steel-cut – sometimes called pinhead or Irish oats. They are whole oat groats that are chewier and have a nutty texture, but be aware they have a longer cooking time than regular oats. You can reduce this by soaking them (in water or milk) overnight. Personally, I tend to use jumbo oats (as seen in my Cherry bakwell overnight oats on p. 125) as they're more easily available but still higher in fibre than regular rolled porridge oats.

- **Soak your grains and seeds:** This can help with digestion and also cuts down on cooking time. You'll notice I recommend soaking the pearl barley overnight for my Soaked pearl barley porridge with kiwi on p. 122 – it means less time in the kitchen and aids nutrient absorption. Soaking chia seeds – see my three chia pudding recipes on p. 128 – creates a mucilage-type of soluble fibre that helps you feel full for longer. Many people find the act of soaking oats for overnight oats (see Cherry bakewell overnight oats on p. 125) also makes them easier to digest.

- **Ferment it:** From sourdough to kefir to sauerkraut, fermenting foods doesn't just improve flavour it can help with nutrition, too. For example, the bacteria used to make sourdough bread help to break down tougher fibres and, in some cases, create more resistant starch. Fermenting can also improve the absorption of minerals such as iron, zinc and magnesium.

You've now got the nuts and bolts of a fibre-friendly life: how to shop, how to swap, how to stack an extra

5g here and there, and how to bring your gut along for the ride without feeling bloated and miserable. You've seen that it doesn't require perfection, just a bit of planning, a few smart store cupboard staples and some gentle consistency (plus the odd fart walk!).

The recipes and meal plans that follow are simply all of this in action. They use the ingredients we've just talked about, the cooking tricks you've picked up in this chapter and the same 'add in, not cut out' approach you've been practising. Think of them as your plug-and-play templates: fibre-rich meals you can lift straight onto your table, then adapt to your own tastes, family commitments, lifestyle and routine.

So now for the fun part: turning all this knowledge into food. In the next section, you'll find breakfasts, lunches, dinners, extras and snacks that put fibre centre-stage without sacrificing comfort, flavour or ease. This is where you start to feel *The Fibre Effect* coming to life – one mouth-watering meal at a time.

Part Two

Fibre On Your Plate

The recipes

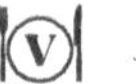 VEGAN

 VEGETARIAN

 FLEXITARIAN

 BATCH-FRIENDLY

CHAPTER 4

Fibre-friendly breakfasts

Whether you eat breakfast the moment you wake or prefer to wait, your first meal is one of the most powerful ways you can set yourself up for the day. A fibre-rich breakfast helps slow the release of glucose into your bloodstream, supports healthy gut motility and fuels your gut microbes so they can start producing those all-important short-chain fatty acids. The result? Steadier energy, better focus, a happier gut and fewer cravings as the day unfolds.

In this chapter, you'll find simple, satisfying recipes designed to deliver plenty of fibre without too much fuss. Many of them can be prepped ahead to make mornings easier – just look for the 'batch-friendly' icon. All the nutritional information under each recipe title – fibre, protein, calories – is listed per serving (toppings are included unless stated otherwise). It has been calculated using reputable nutrition tools but is intended as a guide, not an exact science.

You'll notice lots of Greek yoghurt-based options, as they're versatile, quick and a great source of live bacteria. I tend to use 0% fat Greek yoghurt as many of my clients are looking to manage their energy (calorie) intake and, incidentally, the protein content is higher. Authentic low-fat Greek yoghurt has good levels of calcium, no added sugars and tastes great. Healthy fats are important, which is why I've included plenty of avocados, nuts, seeds, olive oil and oily fish, so you won't be missing out. However, please feel free to swap for full-fat variations if preferred. If you want a plant-based alternative, go for unsweetened soya or coconut yoghurts and you could stir in a little unflavoured vegan protein powder to keep the balance right.

Think of these breakfasts as your fibre-first foundation: delicious, practical and designed to help you feel good all day long.

The recipes at a glance

Soaked Pearl Barley Porridge with Kiwi

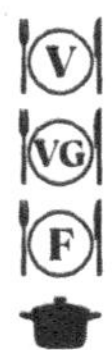

2 SERVINGS

Prep time: 10 mins · Cook time: 20 mins

23g protein · 11g fibre · 370 cals· 8 plants

For the porridge:

» 50g pearl barley
» 400ml milk (I use unsweetened soya milk)
» 2 tbsp wheat bran (or ground flaxseeds)
» ½–1 tsp ground cinnamon to taste
» ¼ tsp ground nutmeg
» 1 banana
» 1 tbsp nut or seed butter

For the topper:

» 2 kiwi fruit, sliced or chopped into small pieces (skin on, if possible!)
» 12 almonds, chopped
» 200g yoghurt of choice (I use 0% fat Greek yoghurt)
» Dusting of ground cinnamon

1. Rinse the pearl barley under running water then place in a lidded container and cover completely with fresh water. Put the lid on and leave to soak overnight in the fridge.
2. In the morning, rinse the barley again under running water and tip into a small saucepan. Add the milk (it'll feel like a lot but don't worry, it'll

all get soaked up by the pearl barley), wheat bran, cinnamon and nutmeg and bring to a simmer over a medium-low heat. Cook for 15–20 minutes, stirring occasionally, until the pearl barley has swelled and is soft and chewy.

3. Meanwhile, mash the banana in a small bowl using a fork, and put to one side.

4. Remove the cooked pearl barley porridge from the heat and stir in the mashed banana and nut (or seed) butter until thoroughly combined.

5. Divide between two bowls and top with the kiwi and chopped almonds, with the Greek yoghurt on the side and dust over some cinnamon. I think the fruit gives it enough sweetness but feel free to add a splash of honey or maple syrup (not included in nutritional breakdown).

TIP: Once cooked, you can decant the porridge into jars and eat cold the following day – like overnight oats. You'll probably need a splash of milk to loosen it before adding the toppings when you're ready to eat. It will keep in the fridge for 2–3 days.

Black Bean and Herb Avocado Toast

2 SERVINGS

Prep time: 5 mins · Cook time: 10 mins

16g protein · 12g fibre · 360 cals · 8+ plants

- » 1 × 400g tin black beans, drained and rinsed
- » 1 tsp olive oil
- » 1 garlic clove, minced
- » 1 tsp ground cumin
- » ½ tsp smoked paprika
- » 1 small avocado
- » 1–2 tsp lime or lemon juice
- » Small handful of coriander, chopped
- » Small handful of basil, chopped
- » Small handful of chives, chopped
- » 2 slices of seeded sourdough bread
- » Optional toppings: chilli flakes, crumbled feta, microgreens (e.g. alfalfa, cress or broccoli sprouts), eggs, grated tempeh or tofu

1. Warm the black beans in a small saucepan with the oil, garlic, cumin and paprika; mash slightly with a fork.
2. In a small bowl, mash the avocado with the lime or lemon juice and herbs, and season with salt and pepper.
3. Toast the bread, spread with the avocado, spoon on the warm beans, and finish with optional herbs or toppings (not included in the nutritional breakdown).

Cherry Bakewell Overnight Oats

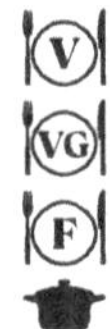

2 SERVINGS

Prep time: 5 mins

20g protein · 11g fibre · 400 cals · 5 plants

- » 60g jumbo oats
- » 2 tbsp ground almonds
- » 2 tbsp chia seeds
- » 200ml milk of choice + a little extra if needed
- » 100g yoghurt of choice (I use 0% fat Greek yoghurt)
- » 2 tsp maple syrup or honey
- » ½ tsp almond extract (optional)
- » 60g cherries (fresh or frozen), halved + 20g to serve
- » 2 tbsp flaked almonds to top

1. Mix the oats, ground almonds, chia seeds, milk, yoghurt, maple syrup and almond extract (if using) in a large jar or bowl. Stir in the 60g cherries. Chill overnight in the fridge – or for at least an hour.
2. Loosen with a little extra milk, if needed, then divide between two bowls (or jars with lids if you are taking them with you). Top equally with the extra cherries and flaked almonds to serve. The oats will keep in the fridge for 3–4 days.

GUT BOOSTER: Add a splash of kefir for some extra live microbes.
FIBRE BOOSTER: Top with some hemp seeds or ground flaxseeds for extra fibre and protein.

Miso Mushrooms on Rye 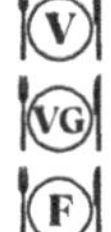

1 SERVING

Prep time: 10 mins · Cook time: 15 mins

11.5g protein · 10g fibre · 430 cals · 6 plants

» 1 tbsp miso paste
» ½ small avocado
» 1 spring onion, thinly sliced
» 200g mushrooms, sliced
» 1 slice of rye bread
» Small handful of parsley, roughly chopped

1. Mix the miso paste with 2 tbsp of water in a small bowl to create a sauce. Leave to one side.
2. In a separate small bowl, mash the avocado with the spring onion (keeping back a few slices of the green part for garnishing).
3. Put a large frying pan on a medium heat (no oil). When hot, add the mushrooms and cook until they've reduced in size and turned golden. Pour over the miso sauce, reduce the heat and allow the sauce to thicken for 1–2 minutes.
4. Toast your rye bread, layer on the avo and spring onion smash and top with the mushrooms. Scatter over the parsley and reserved green spring onion slices.

Cardamom-Spiced Gut-Loving Granola

7 X 50G SERVINGS

Prep time: 10 mins · Cook time: 20 mins

7g protein · 4.5g fibre · 200 cals · 12+ plants

» 150g jumbo oats
» 50g mixed seeds
» 50g mixed nuts, roughly chopped
» 2 tbsp psyllium husk
» 2 tbsp ground flaxseed
» ½ tsp ground cardamom (or cinnamon)
» 2 tbsp coconut oil (or other oil)
» 4 tbsp maple syrup or honey
» 4 level tbsp nut or seed butter

1. Preheat oven to 180°C (160°fan)/350°F.
2. Combine all the dry ingredients in large mixing bowl. Warm the coconut oil, maple syrup and nut or seed butter in a small saucepan on a low heat until the oil has melted (10–20 seconds). Pour the liquid into the dry ingredients and mix well to combine.
3. Tip the mixture onto a baking tray lined with baking parchment. Press the mixture down with the back of a spoon to flatten (this will help create crispy clusters). Bake for 20 minutes or until starting to turn golden.
4. Leave to cool in the tray, then break into clusters. Store in an airtight jar – it will stay fresh for at least a week.

TIP: Add 2 tbsp cacao to the dry ingredients for a chocolate taste and extra fibre.

Chia Pudding Three Ways

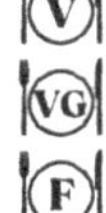

1 SERVING

Prep time: 10 mins

Chocolate hazelnut: 26.5g protein · 13g fibre · 385 cals · 6 plants

Mango and coconut: 24g protein · 11g fibre · 390 cals · 6 plants

Blueberry pie: 26g protein · 11g fibre · 380 cals · 6 plants

For the chia pudding base:

» 1 tbsp chia seeds
» 200ml milk (I use unsweetened soya milk)
» 1 tbsp ground flaxseeds
» 2 tsp maple syrup or honey
» 125g yoghurt of choice (I use 0% fat Greek yoghurt)
» 1 tsp vanilla bean extract (or paste)
» 1 tsp ground cinnamon

Chia pudding base

Put all the ingredients in an airtight container and stir well to combine. Pop on a lid and chill in the fridge overnight or for a minimum of 20 minutes (longer is better) for the chia seeds to swell. When ready to eat, give the mixture a good stir and add a splash of milk to loosen everything up, if needed. Then all you need to do is pick one of the following three options:

Chocolate hazelnut

Stir 1 tbsp (10g) cacao (or cocoa powder) into the chia pudding mixture (add a splash more milk if needed) and top with 10g chopped hazelnuts.

Mango and coconut

Stir 80g chopped mango into the chia pudding mixture (add a splash more milk if needed) and top with 1 tbsp (10g) coconut flakes.

Blueberry pie

Stir 80g blueberries (fresh or frozen) into the chia pudding mixture (add a splash more milk if needed) and top with 10g chopped pistachios.

GUT BOOSTER: Add a splash of kefir to the chia pudding mixture for some extra live microbes.

Smashed Peas and Edamame Beans on Rye

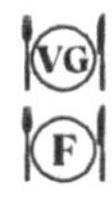

1 SERVING

Prep time: 5 mins · Cook time: 5 mins

26g protein · 10.5g fibre · 395 cals · 4+ plants

- » 65g frozen peas
- » 65g frozen edamame beans
- » 75g cottage cheese
- » 15g feta cheese
- » Squeeze of lemon juice
- » A few fresh mint leaves + extra to serve
- » Pinch of chilli flakes (optional)
- » 1 slice of rye bread

1. Put the peas and edamame beans in a small saucepan of boiling water and cook for 5 minutes, then drain.
2. Mash them in a bowl with the rest of the ingredients, apart from the bread. Taste and season well with pepper.
3. Spoon onto toasted rye bread and scatter over the remaining mint leaves.

Turmeric Kedgeree

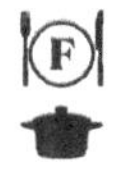

3 SERVINGS

Prep time: 5 mins · Cook time: 15 mins

31g protein · 9.5g fibre · 410 cals · 10 plants

» 1 tbsp olive oil or ghee
» 1 medium onion, finely chopped
» 1 tsp turmeric
» 1 tsp cumin seeds
» 1 tsp mild curry powder
» 1 pouch (250g) cooked brown basmati rice
» ½ x 400g tin green lentils, drained and rinsed
» 150g cooked smoked fish (e.g. haddock or trout), flaked
» Juice of ½ lemon
» 150g frozen peas
» 100g frozen edamame beans
» Large handful (30g) of spinach, chopped
» 3 eggs, hard-boiled and quartered
» Handful of fresh coriander to serve

1. Heat the oil in a large frying pan on a medium heat, and cook the onion until soft. Add the spices, and stir for 1 minute. Stir in the rice and lentils to coat and warm through.
2. Gently fold in the flaked fish with the lemon juice, peas, edamame beans and spinach, and season with salt and pepper. Heat through until the spinach wilts.
3. Serve topped with the egg quarters and coriander.

TIP: The perfect meal for two with leftovers. Keeps in the fridge for 2–3 days.

Maple Pecan Baked Pears

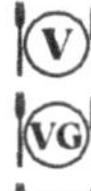

2 SERVINGS

Prep time: 10 mins · Cook time: 40 mins

18g protein · 10g fibre · 380 cals · 10+ plants

» 2 ripe pears
» 2 tbsp jumbo oats
» 1 tbsp ground flaxseeds
» 1 tbsp maple syrup
» 20g pecans, chopped
» 1 tsp vanilla bean extract (or paste)
» 1 tsp ground cinnamon
» ¼ tsp ground nutmeg
» Pinch of salt

To serve:
» 200g yoghurt of choice (I use 0% fat Greek yoghurt)
» 2 tbsp mixed seeds
» Dusting of ground cinnamon

1. Preheat oven to 180°C (160°C fan)/350°F.
2. Slice the pears in half and cut off the stems. Using a teaspoon, scoop out the core and seeds to create space for the filling. Cut a very thin slice off the back of each half so it lies flat without wobbling around.
3. Put the oats, ground flaxseeds, maple syrup, chopped pecans, vanilla, cinnamon, nutmeg and salt into a small bowl and stir to combine well.

4. Place the pears on a baking tray lined with baking parchment. Pile the filling onto the pears and bake for 30–40 minutes or until the pears are soft and the topping is golden.
5. Serve with a dollop of yoghurt, a scattering of mixed seeds and a dusting of cinnamon.

Toasted Rye Porridge with Blackberry Chia Jam

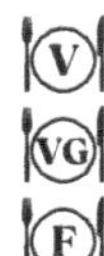

1 SERVING

Prep time: 5 mins · Cook time: 20 mins

27.5g protein · 15.5g fibre · 430 cals · 7+ plants

For the porridge:
» 30g rye flakes
» 200ml milk (I use unsweetened soya milk)
» 1 tsp ground cinnamon
» ¼ tsp ground nutmeg
» 1 heaped tbsp ground flaxseeds
» 125g yoghurt of choice (I use 0% fat Greek yoghurt)

To serve:
» 1 heaped tbsp blackberry chia jam (see p. 210)
» 1 tbsp almond butter (or nut or seed butter of choice)
» 1 tsp maple syrup or honey

1. Start by lightly toasting the rye flakes in a small dry saucepan, being careful not to let them burn – it should only take a minute or so. Stir in the milk, cinnamon and nutmeg and simmer for 10–15 minutes, until the porridge has thickened and the rye flakes are soft and cooked through.
2. Remove from the heat and stir in the flaxseeds and yoghurt until the porridge becomes thick and creamy (this will also cool it down slightly).

3. Spoon into a bowl and top with the blackberry chia jam and drizzle over the almond butter and maple syrup or honey.

TIP: If you haven't got round to making the blackberry chia jam on page 210, swap for 80g blueberries.

Salted Caramel Overnight Oats

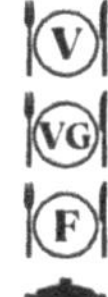

1 SERVING

Prep time: 20 mins

22g protein · 12g fibre · 425 cals · 5 plants

» 30g jumbo oats
» 1 tbsp chia seeds
» 100ml unsweetened soya milk (or milk of choice) + a little extra to loosen
» 80g yoghurt of choice (I use 0% fat Greek yoghurt)
» 5g cacao nibs (or roughly chopped dark chocolate)

For the salted caramel sauce:
» 2 Medjool dates, pitted
» 100ml milk (I use unsweetened soya milk)
» 1 tsp vanilla bean extract (or paste)
» Pinch of flaky sea salt

1. Start by softening the dates, submerging them in a small bowl of boiling water for 5–10 minutes then draining. To make the salted caramel sauce, blend all the ingredients in a food processor until fairly thick. This can take a while, up to 5 minutes. If you are using a Nutribullet, you might want to stop and start it to prevent the motor burning out.
2. Combine the overnight oats ingredients, except the cacao nibs (or dark chocolate), in a glass jar. Pour over the caramel sauce and mix together well. Leave overnight in the fridge or for at least an hour.

3. When ready to eat, loosen with a splash of milk if
    it has thickened, and top with the cacao nibs or
    chocolate.

TIP: It will keep in the fridge for up to 3 days.

Shakshuka with Zhoug 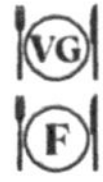

2 SERVINGS

Prep time: 5 mins · Cook time: 30 mins

22g protein · 6g fibre · 550 cals · 10+ plants

For the shakshuka:
» 1 tbsp olive oil
» ½ onion, finely chopped
» 1 red pepper, finely diced
» 100g broccoli, broken into small florets
» 2 garlic cloves, minced
» ½ tsp ground cumin
» ¼ tsp chilli flakes
» 1 × 400g tin plum or chopped tomatoes
» 4 eggs

For the zhoug (this makes extra):
» 1 bunch of coriander (leaves + some tender stems)
» 2 jalapeños
» 2 garlic cloves
» ½ tsp ground cumin
» ½ tsp ground cardamom
» Squeeze of lemon juice
» ½ tsp salt
» 3 tbsp olive oil

To serve:
» 2 tbsp mixed seeds
» Fresh coriander, chopped
» 2 wholemeal pittas

1. To make the zhoug, blitz all the ingredients, adding the oil slowly while the food processor is running, until it forms a thick, spoonable paste.

2. For the shakshuka, heat the oil in a wide pan (a frying pan with a lid works well) on a medium heat, and sauté the onion, pepper, broccoli and garlic until soft. Add the cumin and chilli flakes, and stir for 1 minute. Add the tomatoes, season with salt and pepper, and simmer for 10–12 minutes, until thickened.

3. Make small wells in the sauce and crack in the eggs. Cover and cook gently for 4 minutes, or until the eggs are set to your liking.

4. Top with dollops of zhoug and scatter with mixed seeds and extra herbs. Serve with warm pittas.

CHAPTER 5

Fibre-forward lunches

Lunch is your midday refuel opportunity – to steady your energy, lift your focus and avoid that 3pm slump. A fibre-rich meal does exactly that by slowing digestion, supporting blood sugar balance and feeding the gut microbes that help drive everything from mood to metabolism.

These lunches are built to be satisfying, flavour-packed and genuinely sustaining, with plenty of plants, smart carbs and healthy fats. Many can be prepped ahead or thrown together in minutes, making them ideal for busy days or quick work-from-home meals.

You'll find everything from stuffed pittas and things-on-toast (check out the Miso Beans and Artichoke Hearts on Pesto Toast on p. 154) to crunchy, vibrant salads (Raw Pad Thai on p. 166 is one of my faves) and filling soups like Easy Minestrone Soup on p. 150, through to diversity bowls that practically assemble themselves. Every recipe is deliciously doable and designed to give you a gentle, tasty nudge towards your 30g fibre target.

The recipes at a glance

Crushed Chickpea-Stuffed Pitta

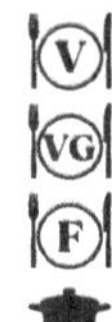

3 SERVINGS

Prep time: 10 mins

18g protein · 11g fibre · 288 cals · 8 plants

- » 1 × 400g tin chickpeas, drained and rinsed
- » 3 heaped tbsp yoghurt of choice (I use 0% fat Greek yoghurt)
- » 2 tsp Dijon or wholegrain mustard
- » 1 small red onion, very finely chopped
- » 1 medium carrot, grated
- » 2 tbsp capers, chopped
- » Small handful of dill, chopped
- » Pinch of sumac
- » 3 wholemeal pittas
- » 3 handfuls of rocket

1. Lightly crush the chickpeas in a bowl with a fork, leaving some texture.
2. Fold in the yoghurt, mustard, red onion, carrot, capers, dill and sumac. Season well with salt and pepper.
3. Toast the pittas, split them open and stuff with rocket and the chickpea mixture.

TIP: Any leftover mixture will keep in the fridge for up to 3 days.

Chicken, Avocado and Quinoa Nourish Bowl

2 SERVINGS

Prep time: 5 mins · Cook time: 5 mins

44g protein · 12.5g fibre · 615 cals · 8 plants

» 1 pouch (200g) cooked quinoa
» ½ × 400g tin chickpeas, drained and rinsed
» 2 small cooked chicken breasts (200g in total), sliced or shredded
» 8 radishes, chopped
» 1 small avocado, diced
» 40g broccoli sprouts
» 3 tbsp sauerkraut

For the herb dressing:
» 2 tbsp olive oil
» 1 tbsp lemon juice
» 1 small garlic clove, grated
» 2 tsp Dijon mustard
» 1 tsp maple syrup or honey
» Handful of parsley, finely chopped

1. To make the herb dressing, whisk all the ingredients in a small bowl until well combined. Set to one side.
2. Warm the quinoa and chickpeas in a small saucepan and season lightly with salt and pepper. Divide between two bowls, then build each one by layering on the chicken, radishes, avocado, broccoli sprouts

and sauerkraut. Pour over the dressing and toss to combine everything together.

TIP: If you are meal prepping, don't dress the salad until ready to eat. The nourish bowls will keep in the fridge for up to 3 days.

Coconut Lentils with Crispy Kale

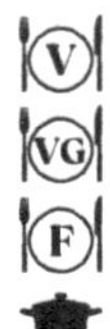

4 SERVINGS

Prep time: 15 mins · Cook time: 30 mins

17g protein · 12.5g fibre · 440 cals · 10+ plants

- » 1 tbsp coconut oil
- » 1 medium onion, finely chopped
- » Pinch of salt
- » 3 garlic cloves, minced
- » 1 thumb-sized piece of fresh ginger, grated
- » 1 tsp cumin seeds
- » 1 tsp mustard seeds
- » 1 tsp turmeric
- » 2 tsp garam masala
- » 200g dried red lentils, rinsed
- » 3 medium-sized firm tomatoes, grated
- » 1 × 400ml tin full-fat coconut milk
- » 500ml stock or water
- » Juice of 1 small lemon
- » Handful of coriander leaves to garnish
- » 1 green chilli, seeds removed and finely chopped (optional)

For the crispy kale:
- » 200g curly kale (or cavolo nero)
- » 1 tbsp olive oil

1. Preheat oven to 180°C (160°C fan)/350°F.
2. Heat the coconut oil in a large saucepan on a medium-low heat and soften the onion with a pinch of salt for 5–8 minutes. Stir in the garlic, ginger and spices and cook for a further 1–2 minutes.
3. Add the lentils, grated tomatoes, coconut milk and stock. Bring to a low boil, then turn down the heat and simmer for 20 minutes until thickened. Season with salt and pepper, to taste.
4. Meanwhile, wash the kale and dry it thoroughly. It needs to be completely dry to ensure it crisps up in the oven. Remove the stalks and slice the leaves into small pieces. Toss the leaves in the olive oil and a pinch of salt. Arrange in a single layer on a baking tray and cook in the oven for 10 minutes, until crisp, checking on them occasionally to make sure they're not burning.
5. Spoon the lentils into bowls, squeeze over the lemon juice and top with the coriander, crispy kale and green chilli (if using).

TIP: Add some crispy tofu, shredded chicken or even boiled eggs to up the protein.

Crispy Chilli Oil Buckwheat Noodles

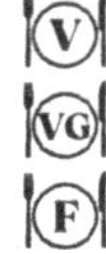

2 SERVINGS

Prep time: 5 mins · Cook time: 20 mins
31.5g protein · 10g fibre · 515 cals · 6 plants

» 150g buckwheat soba noodles
» 150g tempeh, grated
» 1 tbsp crispy chilli oil (more if you like spice)
» 2 garlic cloves, grated
» 1 red pepper, thinly sliced (or any other veg)
» 3 spring onions, sliced
» 1 tbsp soy sauce
» 2 tsp sesame seeds to serve

1. Cook the noodles according to the packet instructions. Drain, reserving a splash of cooking water.
2. In a medium frying pan, fry the grated tempeh in the crispy chilli oil for about 10 minutes or until golden. Add the garlic, red pepper, spring onions and soy sauce and cook for a further 5–8 minutes to soften the red pepper.
3. Toss in the noodles, loosening with the reserved noodle water, if needed. Scatter over the sesame seeds to serve.

TIP: Crispy chilli oil (also known as chilli crisp or chilli crunch) is widely sold in supermarkets – you'll probably find it in the Asian or World Food section.

Halloumi Power Bowl with Figs and Honey-Lemon Dressing

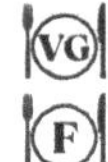

2 SERVINGS

Prep time: 5 mins · Cook time: 8 mins

25g protein · 11g fibre · 535 cals · 8+ plants

- » 100g halloumi, sliced
- » 1 pouch (250g) cooked freekeh or bulgur wheat
- » 80g watercress or mixed leafy greens
- » 2 fresh figs, sliced
- » Small handful of fresh mint
- » 2 tbsp mixed seeds

For the dressing:
- » 1 tbsp olive oil
- » ½ tbsp lemon juice
- » 1 tsp honey

1. To make the dressing, whisk together all the ingredients in a small bowl.
2. Heat a small frying pan on a medium heat (no oil required) and cook the halloumi slices for 5–8 minutes, turning them over, until golden on both sides.
3. Now build the bowl, adding the freekeh or bulgur wheat and then layering on the watercress or mixed leafy greens, halloumi, figs, mint and mixed seeds. Spoon over the dressing just before serving.

Easy Minestrone Soup

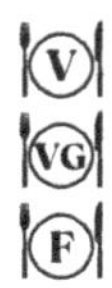

4 SERVINGS

Prep time: 5 mins · Cook time: 30 mins

15g protein · 11g fibre · 400 cals · 10+ plants

- » 2 tbsp olive oil
- » 200g soffritto mix (or 1 onion, 1 celery stick and 1 carrot, all finely diced)
- » A pinch of salt
- » 1 leek, sliced
- » 1 medium courgette, grated
- » 1 × 400g tin chopped tomatoes
- » 1–1.5 litres vegetable stock
- » ½ tsp dried oregano
- » 30g Parmesan and the rind, if available (or vegetarian hard cheese/3 tbsp nutritional yeast)
- » 150g wholewheat pasta (tiny shapes)
- » 1 × 400g tin cannellini beans, drained and rinsed
- » 150g frozen peas
- » 4 slices of seeded sourdough bread, toasted

1. Heat the oil in a large saucepan on a low heat and cook the onion, celery and carrot with a generous pinch of salt for 8–10 minutes, until soft.
2. Add the leek, courgette, tomatoes, 1 litre of stock, oregano and Parmesan rind, if available, bring to the boil, then turn down to a low heat and simmer for 10–12 minutes.
3. Stir in the pasta, beans and peas and cook for 5–10 minutes, or until the pasta is tender. Add more stock if it starts to look too thick.

4. Season with salt and pepper and serve with grated Parmesan (or vegetarian hard cheese/nutritional yeast) and toasted sourdough.

TIP: The minestrone will keep in the fridge for 3–4 days.

Leek, Broccoli and Potato Soup with Fennel and Miso

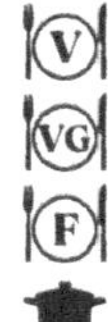

4 SERVINGS

Prep time: 10 mins · Cook time: 30 mins

Without beans: 12.5g protein · 9g fibre · 313 cals · 9+ plants

With crispy garlic beans (see p. 204 for recipe): 16.5g protein · 13g fibre · 400 cals · 10+ plants

» 2 tbsp olive oil
» 1 large leek, sliced
» 1 celery stick, sliced
» Pinch of salt
» 300g potatoes, peeled and cubed
» ½ bulb of fennel, roughly chopped
» 1 tbsp grated fresh ginger
» 1 litre vegetable stock
» 250g broccoli florets
» 150g frozen peas
» 2 large handfuls of spinach
» 1 tbsp white miso

To serve:
» 4 heaped tbsp yoghurt of choice (I use 0% fat Greek yoghurt)
» Cracked black pepper
» Crispy garlic beans (see p. 204) (optional)
» 4 slices of seeded sourdough bread, toasted

1. Heat the oil in a large saucepan on a medium heat. Add the leek and celery with a generous pinch of salt and cook for 8–10 minutes, until soft.
2. Add the potatoes, fennel and ginger, stir well and cook for 2 minutes. Pour in the stock and simmer for 12–15 minutes, until the potato is soft.
3. Add the broccoli, peas and spinach and cook for 3–4 minutes; don't overcook the greens to keep their lovely bright colour.
4. Remove from the heat and stir in the miso. Blend fully or partially, depending on your preference.
5. Serve topped with the yoghurt, plenty of cracked black pepper and the crispy beans on p. 204 (if using), plus some toasted sourdough on the side.

TIP: If you haven't got round to making the crispy beans, a tbsp of pumpkin seeds would make a good alternative.

Miso Beans and Artichoke Hearts on Pesto Toast

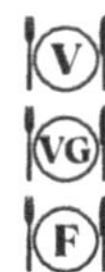

2 SERVINGS

Prep time: 5 mins · Cook time: 10 mins

15g protein · 10g fibre · 450 cals · 8+ plants

» 2 tsp olive oil
» 1 small shallot or 2 spring onions, finely sliced
» 6 artichoke hearts from a jar, drained and sliced
» 1 garlic clove, minced
» 1 × 400g tin butter beans, drained and rinsed
» 1 tsp miso paste
» 2 handfuls of spinach
» 2 slices of seeded sourdough bread
» 2 tbsp pesto
» 2 tbsp mixed seeds
» Small handful of chives, snipped into small pieces
  using scissors

1. In a medium frying pan, heat the oil and gently fry
   the shallot (or spring onions), artichokes and garlic
   for 5 minutes.
2. Add the beans and warm them through – adding a
   splash of warm water if it all feels a little dry.
3. Stir in the miso and then the spinach, until it has
   just wilted.
4. Toast the sourdough and spread with the pesto.
   Pile the beans on top, and finish with the mixed
   seeds and chopped chives.

Pesto Orzo Salad

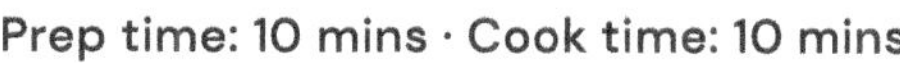

3 SERVINGS

Prep time: 10 mins · Cook time: 10 mins

With regular orzo: 20g protein · 10.5g fibre · 515 cals · 5 plants

With chickpea orzo: 25g protein · 14.5g fibre · 515 cals ·

6 plants

» 200g dried orzo (regular or chickpea)
» 3 tbsp pesto
» 1 × 400g tin chickpeas, drained and rinsed
» 120g cherry tomatoes, halved
» 60g sun-dried tomatoes, chopped
» Juice of ½ lemon
» 60g rocket
» 2 tbsp toasted pine nuts

1. Cook the orzo according to the packet instructions, then drain well.
2. In a serving bowl, toss the warm orzo with the pesto. Fold in the chickpeas and both types of tomatoes. Season with lemon juice, salt and pepper.
3. Stir through the rocket just before serving and top with the pine nuts.

TIP: This salad is perfect for meal prep and will keep for up to 3 days in the fridge – add the rocket just before eating so it doesn't go soggy.

Pea and Mint Soup

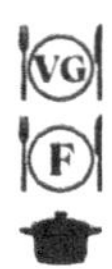

4 SERVINGS

Prep time: 10 mins · Cook time: 30 mins

24g protein · 10.5g fibre · 365 cals · 8+ plants

» 1 tbsp olive oil
» 1 medium onion, roughly chopped
» 3 celery sticks, sliced
» 4 garlic cloves, halved
» 400g frozen peas
» 1 x 400g tin white beans (I used butter beans), drained and rinsed
» 800ml vegetable stock
» 150g spinach
» Small handful of mint leaves (keep a few back for garnishing)
» 250g block of halloumi, cut into small cubes
» 2 tsp garlic granules (optional)
» 4 slices of sourdough bread, toasted
» Sprinkle of chilli flakes to serve

1. Heat the oil in a medium saucepan and gently fry the onion, celery and garlic, until softened. Add the peas, beans and 600ml of the stock (keep the remaining 200ml to one side to add if things start to look like they need loosening). Bring to the boil, then turn down the heat and simmer for 10 minutes.

2. Add the spinach and mint leaves, just until they wilt, then take off the heat and blend with a stick blender. Season, to taste, with salt and pepper.

3. Fry the halloumi cubes in a hot dry frying pan (you can sprinkle them with garlic granules if you have some), turning each cube over until they are browned on all sides. Keep an eye on them and move them around the pan frequently, as they can go from brown to burnt quite quickly. Turn the heat down once they start to get some colour.

4. Serve the soup with the toasted sourdough, a sprinkle of mint leaves and chilli flakes and topped with the halloumi 'croutons'.

TIP: Swap the halloumi for roasted chickpeas for a vegan option and extra plant points.

Tomato and Red Pepper Pearl Barley Risotto 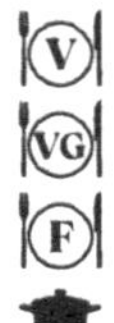

4 SERVINGS

Prep time: 15 mins · Cook time: 1 hour 10 mins

15g protein · 10g fibre · 470 cals · 10+ plants

» 2 red peppers, cut into chunks
» 300g cherry tomatoes
» 3 tbsp olive oil
» ½ tsp dried oregano
» A pinch of salt
» 4 tbsp mixed seeds
» 1 red onion, finely chopped
» 3 garlic cloves, sliced
» 200g pearl barley, rinsed
» 1 tbsp tomato purée
» 800–900ml hot vegetable stock
» 50g Parmesan, grated (or vegetarian hard cheese/ 3 tbsp nutritional yeast)

1. Preheat oven to 230°C (210°C fan)/410°F. Put the peppers and tomatoes on a baking tray and toss to coat in 2 tbsp of the oil, the oregano and a generous pinch of salt. Roast in the oven for 25–30 minutes, until everything has softened and the tomatoes are starting to blister.
2. Meanwhile, toast the seeds in a small dry frying pan on a medium heat for a few minutes until they turn golden, being careful not to burn them. Tip onto a plate.

3. Blitz the roasted veg in a blender until smooth.

4. In a deep wide saucepan on a medium heat, soften the onion and garlic in the remaining 1 tbsp oil. Stir in the barley and tomato purée for 1 minute. Gradually pour in 800ml of the hot stock, stirring until fully absorbed before adding more. Cook until the barley is tender – it will take around 30 minutes.

5. Stir in the roasted vegetable purée, loosening with more stock if needed.

6. Finish with the grated Parmesan (or vegetarian hard cheese/3 tbsp nutritional yeast), some black pepper and the toasted seeds.

TIP: To top up the protein, serve with pan-fried white fish, crispy tempeh or baked feta.

Sweet Potato with Freekeh and Whipped Tahini

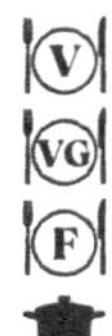

2 SERVINGS

Prep time: 10 mins · Cook time: 35 mins

20g protein · 12.5g fibre · 460 cals · 12+ plants

» 2 medium (130g each) sweet potatoes, halved lengthways
» ½ tbsp olive oil
» 2 tsp mix of spices (e.g. paprika, ground cumin and chilli)
» 1 pouch (200g) cooked freekeh
» 2 large handfuls (40g in total) of rocket
» 20g pomegranate seeds
» 2 tbsp chopped parsley
» 2 tbsp mixed seeds

For the whipped tahini:
» 2 tbsp tahini
» 2–3 tbsp warm water
» Juice of ½ lemon
» 1 garlic clove, smashed

1. Preheat oven to 200°C (180°C fan)/400°F. Place the sweet potato halves in a roasting tray and rub to coat in the oil and spices. Cook for 30–35 minutes, until they start to char around the edges and are cooked all the way through.

2. In a small bowl, whisk the tahini with the warm water, lemon juice, garlic and some salt and pepper to a thick, creamy consistency.
3. Serve the roasted sweet potatoes in two bowls and top with the freekeh, rocket, whipped tahini, pomegranate seeds, parsley and mixed seeds. Season as needed.

TIP: Add in some flaked mackerel, tofu or a sprinkling of feta to easily top up the protein.

One-Pot Creamy White Beans

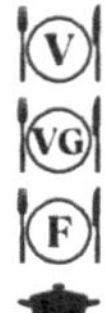

4 SERVINGS

Prep time: 10 mins · Cook time: 25 mins

16g protein · 11g fibre · 415 cals · 10+ plants

» 1 tbsp olive oil
» 200g frozen soffritto mix (or 1 large onion, 2 large carrots and 2 celery sticks, all finely chopped)
» Pinch of salt
» 4 large garlic cloves, minced
» 1 tsp dried oregano
» 2 tbsp tomato purée
» 2 x 400g tins (or 1 x 700g jar) of white beans (e.g. butter beans, cannellini beans, haricot beans etc.), drained and rinsed
» 1 x 400g tin chopped tomatoes
» 200ml vegetable stock
» 20g nutritional yeast (or 60g Parmesan/vegetarian hard cheese, grated)
» Large handful of spinach leaves, finely chopped
» Small handful of basil, finely chopped
» 200ml full-fat coconut milk (or vegan cream)
» Rocket or mixed salad leaves to serve
» 4 slices of seeded sourdough bread, toasted

1. In a large heavy-bottomed pan, heat the oil on a medium-to-low heat. Add the soffritto mix and a generous pinch of salt and cook for 10 minutes, stirring occasionally, until softened.

2. Add the garlic and oregano and cook for 2 minutes, then add the tomato purée and cook for a further 2 minutes. Tip in the beans, tomatoes and stock, and stir well. Turn up the heat until everything starts to bubble, then reduce the heat and simmer for 5–10 minutes until the sauce thickens. Taste and season with salt and pepper.

3. Add the nutritional yeast (or Parmesan/vegetarian hard cheese), spinach and basil and stir for a couple of minutes, until the spinach wilts. Turn off the heat and pour in the coconut milk (or vegan cream). Stir to mix through thoroughly.

4. Spoon into large bowls and serve with a handful of rocket or mixed leaves on the side together with the toasted sourdough.

Warm Winter Nourish Bowl

3 SERVINGS

Prep time: 10 mins · Cook time: 30 mins

23g protein · 17g fibre · 520 cals · 10+ plants

» 1 small cauliflower (around 500g), cut into thick slices
» 1 × 400g tin chickpeas, drained, rinsed and patted dry
» 1 tbsp olive oil
» 1 tsp paprika
» 1 tsp ground cumin
» ¼ tsp ground cinnamon
» ¼ tsp ground ginger
» 1 tsp garlic granules
» 2 tsp apple cider vinegar
» 1 pouch (250g) cooked quinoa
» 50g finely chopped parsley
» 50g finely chopped spinach
» 3 medium tomatoes, finely diced
» ½ cucumber, finely diced
» 1 small red onion, finely diced

For the dressing:
» 2 tbsp lemon juice
» 1 tbsp olive oil
» 2 tbsp tahini
» 1 garlic clove, minced
» Pinch of chilli flakes
» 2 tbsp warm water

To serve:

» 3 tbsp pomegranate seeds
» 3 tsp dukkah

1. Preheat oven to 210°C (190°C fan)/375°F.
2. On a large baking tray, toss the cauliflower and chickpeas with the oil, spices, garlic granules and apple
   cider vinegar and season well with salt and pepper.
   Roast for 25–30 minutes, until crisp and golden.
   Allow to cool slightly and then, using a large knife,
   chop the cauliflower into very small pieces. Set to
   one side.
3. Make the dressing by whisking together all the
   ingredients in a small bowl until smooth.
4. In a medium-sized bowl, toss the cooked quinoa
   with the finely chopped cauliflower and chickpeas
   and the chopped tomatoes, cucumber, spinach,
   parsley and red onion. Spoon into serving bowls,
   fold through the dressing, then top with the pomegranate seeds and sprinkle over the dukkah to serve.

TIP: It will keep for up to 3 days in the fridge. It's also
really nice with crispy tofu, shredded chicken or flaked
mackerel if you want to bump up the protein further.

Raw Pad Thai

2 SERVINGS

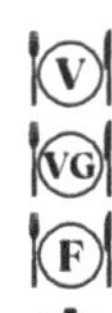

Prep time: 10 mins

15g protein · 10g fibre · 420 cals · 8+ plants

» 250g spiralised courgette
» 350g mix of veg (e.g. cabbage, carrot, cucumber, peppers, sugar snaps, mange tout and spring onion), julienned
» Large handful of beansprouts
» 1 red chilli, sliced
» 40g crushed peanuts to serve
» Lime wedges to serve

For the satay dressing:
» 2 tbsp crunchy peanut butter
» 1 tsp sesame oil
» 2 tbsp soy sauce
» 1–2 tbsp lime juice
» 1–2 tsp honey or maple syrup
» Warm water to loosen

1. Make the satay dressing by whisking all the ingredients together in a small bowl until smooth and well combined. Loosen with a little warm water, if needed.
2. In a large bowl, toss all the veg in the dressing just before serving. Top with the chilli, peanuts and a squeeze of lime.

CHAPTER 6

Fibre-fuelled dinners

Dinner is where everything you've learned about fibre comes together on the plate: the flavours, the nourishment, the diversity and the effortless habits that make this way of eating stick. These recipes are designed to be colourful, satisfying and deeply delicious, but also practical enough for real life. Think quick 20-minute midweek meals, cosy one-pan dishes, vibrant tray bakes and Friday-night feasts that feel comforting without leaving you sluggish.

Across this chapter you'll find pastas boosted with legumes and greens, a hearty dahl, loaded tray bakes, grain bowls and bold bean dishes. Many can be doubled for batch cooking or halved if you're flying solo, and most use affordable, everyday fibre heroes you already know from the earlier chapters.

As you cook your way through Cavolo Nero Anchovy Linguine on p. 194, Beef and Beetroot Koftas with Whipped Feta on p.176, Veg-Squeezed Mac and Cheese on p. 182, Borlotti Bean Ragú on p. 180 and the rest, you'll see the same principles repeated: plant diversity, smart shortcuts, plenty of taste and those small fibre-boosting tweaks that make a big difference over time.

Whether you're after fast, family-friendly, budget-friendly or something a bit special, these are the meals that help you end the day feeling well-fed and quietly confident you're doing something good for your health.

The recipes at a glance

Quick Ribollita

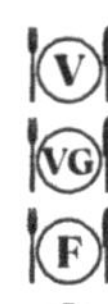

4 SERVINGS

Prep time: 10 mins · Cook time: 25 mins

18g protein · 10.5g fibre · 440 cals · 9 plants

» 1 tbsp olive oil
» 1 medium onion, finely diced
» 1 carrot, finely diced
» 1 celery stick, finely diced
» 200g cavolo nero, stalks removed and roughly chopped
» 2 garlic cloves, finely chopped
» 4 medium tomatoes, grated
» 1 litre vegetable stock
» 1 tsp dried rosemary
» 60g Parmesan, grated (add the rind to the pot if you have it) or vegetarian hard cheese
» 1 × 400g tin haricot beans, drained and rinsed
» 4 tbsp pumpkin seeds
» Pinch of chilli flakes to serve (optional)
» 4 slices of seeded sourdough bread, toasted

1. Heat the oil in a large saucepan on a low heat and gently cook the onion, carrot and celery, with the lid on, for 5 minutes. Remove the lid and add the cavolo nero and garlic. Increase the heat to medium and cook for 3 minutes, until the garlic is slightly coloured.

2. Stir in the tomatoes for 2 minutes. Add the stock, rosemary and the Parmesan rind if you have it. Simmer on a low heat for 10 minutes.

3. Add the beans and warm through for 5 minutes. Season, to taste, with salt and pepper.

4. Serve in bowls, scattered with the grated Parmesan or vegetarian hard cheese, pumpkin seeds and chilli flakes (if using) with the toasted sourdough on the side.

TIP: Add ricotta or grated fried tofu or tempeh to increase the protein. See the Greens and beans taco salad recipe on p. 188 for instructions on how to fry grated tofu and/or tempeh.

Broccoli Fried Rice with Crispy Egg

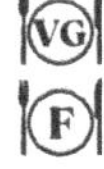

2 SERVINGS

Prep time: 5 mins · Cook time: 15 mins

17g protein · 10g fibre · 280 cals · 7 plants

» 1 tbsp olive oil + extra to fry the eggs
» 2 garlic cloves, minced
» 1cm fresh ginger, minced
» ½ tsp dried chilli flakes or 1 red chilli, deseeded and finely chopped
» 300g 'rice' made from blitzed (or grated) broccoli
» 150g mixed crunchy veg (e.g. sugar snap peas, mange tout, carrot, peppers), all finely sliced
» 2 tbsp soy sauce
» 3 spring onions, sliced

To serve:
» 2 eggs
» 2 tsp black sesame seeds
» 2 tsp crispy chilli oil

1. Heat the oil in a medium frying pan and cook the garlic, ginger and chilli for 1–2 minutes, until softened but not to the point where they start to brown. Add the broccoli 'rice' and mixed veg, and stir-fry for 4–5 minutes, until the broccoli is cooked through.
2. Add the soy sauce and spring onion, and stir-fry until the onion softens. At the same time, fry the

eggs in a separate frying pan with a little olive oil, to your liking.

3. Divide between two bowls, topping the broccoli fried 'rice' with a crispy fried egg, sesame seeds and crispy chilli oil to serve.

50:50 Spag Bol (half beef, half lentils)

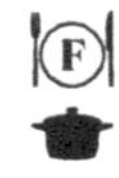

Prep time: 10 mins · Cook time: 1 hour

31g protein · 16.5g fibre · 490 cals · 8+ plants

- » 1 tbsp olive oil
- » 1 large onion, finely diced
- » 1 large carrot, finely diced
- » 1 large celery stick, finely diced
- » 2 garlic cloves, minced
- » 250g lean beef or turkey mince (or 300g Quorn mince)
- » 1 tbsp tomato purée
- » 1 x 400g tin cooked lentils, drained and rinsed
- » 1 × 400g tin chopped tomatoes
- » 200–300ml stock or water
- » 2 rosemary sprigs
- » ½ tsp dried oregano
- » 300g wholewheat spaghetti

1. In a large frying pan, heat the oil and gently cook the diced onion, carrot and celery for 10 minutes, until soft. Add the garlic and cook for 1 minute.
2. Increase the heat and add the mince. Cook until well browned, breaking it up as it cooks with a wooden spoon.
3. Stir in the tomato purée, lentils, tomatoes, 200ml of the stock, rosemary and oregano. Bring to

a simmer, cover with a lid and cook on low for 45 minutes. Add the remaining stock if it looks like it needs loosening a little.

4. Cook the spaghetti in a large pan of salted boiling water according to the packet instructions.

5. Remove the rosemary sprigs from the bolognese, season generously with salt and black pepper, then toss with the drained spaghetti.

Beef and Beetroot Koftas with Whipped Feta 

4 SERVINGS

Prep time: 15 mins · Cook time: 20 mins

35g protein · 10g fibre · 500 cals · 10+ plants

» 300g lean beef mince
» 1 pouch (200g) cooked lentils
» 1 raw beetroot, peeled and finely grated
» 1 onion, grated or very finely chopped
» 2 garlic cloves, crushed
» 1 tsp ground cumin
» ½ tsp smoked paprika
» 1 tsp dried mint
» 2 tbsp chopped parsley
» Drizzle of olive oil

For the whipped feta:
» 150g feta
» 3 tbsp yoghurt of choice (I use 0% fat Greek yoghurt)
» 1 tbsp olive oil
» Juice of ½ lemon
» A few grinds of freshly ground black pepper

To serve:
» 4 wholemeal pitas
» Large handful of salad leaves or shredded lettuce
» ⅓ cucumber, sliced
» 1 large tomato, sliced
» 1 small red onion, sliced

1. Preheat oven to 160°C (140°C fan)/320°F.

2. In a large bowl, mix together the beef mince, lentils, beetroot, onion, garlic, cumin, paprika, mint and parsley, and season generously with salt and pepper. Combine well and shape into 12 koftas or oval patties.

3. Drizzle the oil in a frying pan on a medium heat and cook the koftas or patties for 3–4 minutes on each side, until browned and cooked through. If you need to do them in batches, you can keep them warm in the oven on a low heat.

4. Meanwhile, blend or mash the feta with the yoghurt, oil, lemon juice and black pepper, until smooth and creamy.

5. Toast the pitas and split them open. Spread with the whipped feta, add the koftas (or patties) and stuff with the salad.

Black Bean Burger

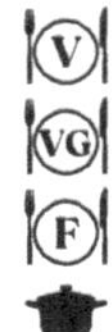

4 SERVINGS

Prep time: 20 mins · Cook time: 15 mins

25g protein · 12g fibre · 575 cals · 8+ plants

» 50g walnuts (or toasted walnuts, finely chopped)
» 1 × 400g tin black beans, drained, rinsed and dried very well with paper towel
» 100g cooked quinoa
» 1 small red onion, finely chopped
» 1 large egg, lightly whisked
» 1 tsp garlic granules
» 1 tsp ground cumin
» 1 tsp smoked paprika
» 40g panko breadcrumbs
» 3 tbsp BBQ sauce
» 2 tbsp chopped coriander stalks
» 4 slices (25g each) Cheddar or vegan cheese

For the burger sauce:
» 1 small avocado
» 2 tbsp yoghurt of choice (I use 0% fat Greek yoghurt)
» Small handful of coriander leaves, finely chopped
» 1 clove of raw garlic, minced
» Juice of 1 lime

To serve:
» 4 burger buns
» Handful of lettuce
» 1 large tomato, sliced

1. Toast the walnuts in a hot dry frying pan for a few
   minutes until they turn golden and give off a rich,
   nutty aroma, being careful not to let them burn.
   Tip onto a plate to cool, then chop finely.
2. In a medium bowl, roughly mash the beans. Mix
   in the cooked quinoa, onion, egg, garlic granules,
   spices, panko breadcrumbs, walnuts, BBQ sauce
   and coriander stalks.
3. Using slightly wet hands, shape the mixture into
   4 patties. Chill in the fridge for 20 minutes (or
   overnight if you're planning ahead) to 'set'.
4. Meanwhile, mash all the burger sauce ingredients
   together in a small bowl and set to one side.
5. Pan-fry each burger in a few sprays of olive oil on a
   low heat for 3 minutes on each side, until they start
   to crisp up on the outside and are hot all the way
   through. Top each burger with a slice of Cheddar
   or vegan cheese and leave in the pan (cover with a
   lid if you have one) until the cheese melts.
6. To assemble the burgers, spread the bottom half
   of each bun with the sauce, top with some lettuce,
   the burger and cheese, a slice of tomato and the
   bun lid.

Borlotti Bean Ragú (beef or Quorn)

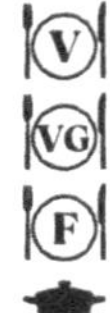

4 SERVINGS

Prep time: 15 mins · Cook time: 45 mins

With beef: 45.5g protein · 19g fibre · 390 cals · 10+ plants

With Quorn: 42.5g protein · 25g fibre · 375 cals · 10+ plants

» 1 tbsp olive oil
» 1 onion, finely chopped
» 1 carrot, finely diced
» 1 celery stick, finely diced
» 200g mushrooms, finely chopped
» Pinch of salt
» 300g lean beef or Quorn mince
» 1 × 400g tin chopped tomatoes
» 1 × 400g tin borlotti beans, drained and rinsed
» 1 tsp mixed dried herbs
» 200g mung bean tagliatelle (or pasta of choice)
» 20g grated Parmesan (or vegetarian hard cheese/ nutritional yeast)
» Handful of basil, roughly torn, to finish
» Pinch of chilli flakes (optional)

1. Heat the oil in a large frying pan on a medium-low heat and gently cook the onion, carrot, celery and mushrooms with a generous pinch of salt, until soft.
2. Increase the heat and add the mince. Cook until well browned, breaking it up with a wooden spoon as you go.

3. Add the tomatoes, beans and mixed dried herbs. Lower the heat and simmer for 20–25 minutes until it starts to thicken.
4. Cook the pasta according to the packet instructions.
5. Season the ragú generously with salt and pepper. Serve over the drained pasta with the Parmesan (or vegetarian hard cheese/nutritional yeast), torn basil and chilli flakes if you like a bit of heat.

TIP: The ragú will keep in the fridge for up to 3 days.

Veg-Squeezed Mac and Cheese

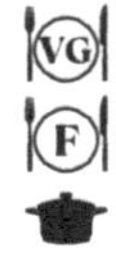

4 SERVINGS

Prep time: 15 mins · Cook time: 1 hour

21.5g protein · 12g fibre · 500 cals · 8+ plants

» 300g butternut squash, seeds removed, cut into smallish chunks
» 1 tbsp olive oil
» 175g wholewheat macaroni or any small legume pasta
» 150g small broccoli florets
» 2 garlic cloves, crushed
» 1 tsp mustard (any type)
» 1 tsp white miso
» 1 x 400g tin cannellini beans, drained and rinsed
» 100–200ml vegetable stock (to loosen the béchamel sauce)
» 100g spinach
» 80g Cheddar, grated
» 50g breadcrumbs
» Mixed salad leaves to serve

For the béchamel sauce:
» 40g butter
» 40g plain wholemeal flour
» 400ml milk (of your choice)

1. Preheat oven to 200°C (180°C fan)/400°F. In a roasting tin, drizzle the butternut squash chunks with the oil and cook in the oven for 30–40 minutes, until tender.

2. While the butternut squash is cooking, make the béchamel sauce. In a large saucepan, melt the butter on a low-to-medium heat. Stir in the flour gradually, whisking constantly to form a smooth paste. Continue cooking the paste for 1–2 minutes, stirring continuously; this cooks out the raw flour taste, but be careful not to let it brown. Remove the pan from the heat and gradually whisk in the milk, a little at a time. Whisk fairly vigorously after each addition to avoid lumps. Once all the milk has been added and the mixture is smooth, return the pan to a medium-low heat. Bring to a gentle simmer for 5–10 minutes, whisking frequently, until the sauce thickens. Turn off the heat.

3. Meanwhile, in a large saucepan, cook the macaroni (or legume pasta) according to the packet instructions. While it is cooking, place a colander or metal sieve on top of the saucepan and put the broccoli in it. Put the lid on top and lightly steam the broccoli for 5 minutes.

4. Remove the squash from the oven and tip it into the saucepan with the béchamel sauce. Add the garlic, mustard, miso and beans and then, using a stick blender, blend everything together. Use a little stock to loosen the sauce if it is too thick.

5. In the same roasting tin you used to cook the butternut squash, combine the cooked, drained,

macaroni (or legume pasta) with the béchamel sauce, spinach and steamed broccoli, and season with salt and pepper. Give it a good mix and top with the grated Cheddar and breadcrumbs, then bake for 20 minutes until bubbling. Serve with mixed salad leaves on the side.

TIP: It will keep for 3–4 days in the fridge.

Cheesy Green Orzo Bake 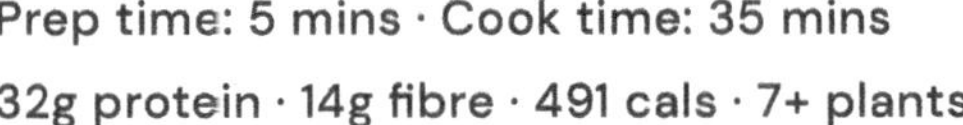

4 SERVINGS

Prep time: 5 mins · Cook time: 35 mins

32g protein · 14g fibre · 491 cals · 7+ plants

- » 1 tbsp olive oil
- » 1 leek, sliced
- » Pinch of salt
- » 250g chickpea orzo
- » 250g broccoli florets
- » 2 large handfuls of kale or spinach, chopped
- » 120g frozen peas
- » 1 × 400g tin cannellini or haricot beans, drained and rinsed
- » 500ml vegetable stock
- » 150g Cheddar, grated
- » 4 large handfuls of mixed salad leaves to serve

1. Preheat oven to 180°C (160°C fan)/350°F.
2. Heat the oil in a large deep pan on a medium heat. Sauté the leek with a generous pinch of salt until soft.
3. Add the orzo, broccoli, kale or spinach, peas, beans, stock and two-thirds (100g) of the grated cheese. Mix together, then transfer to a large baking dish.
4. Cover the dish with foil and bake for 20 minutes, then uncover, top with the remaining cheese and bake for 6–8 minutes, until melted and bubbling. Rest for 5 minutes before serving with a large handful of mixed salad leaves on the side.

TIP: The orzo bake will keep in the fridge for 3-4 days.

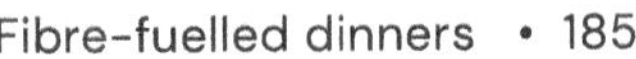

Dahl with Roasted Carrots and Egg

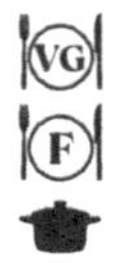

4 SERVINGS

Prep time: 15 mins · Cook time: 45 mins

25g protein · 10g fibre · 345 cals · 12+ plants

- » 4 large carrots, cut in half lengthways
- » 1 tbsp olive oil
- » 1 tbsp coconut oil
- » 1 onion, finely chopped
- » Pinch of salt
- » 3 garlic cloves, grated
- » 2cm fresh ginger, grated
- » 1 tsp turmeric
- » 1 tsp ground coriander
- » 1 tsp cumin seeds
- » 2 tsp garam masala
- » Pinch of ground cinnamon
- » 3 medium tomatoes, grated
- » 1 green chilli, sliced
- » 250g dried yellow split peas
- » 750ml–1 litre stock of your choice

To serve:
- » 4 eggs
- » Juice of ½ lemon
- » Handful of coriander leaves
- » Drizzle of chilli oil (optional)

1. Heat oven to 200°C (180°C fan)/400°F.

2. Put the halved carrots on a small baking tray, drizzle with the olive oil and season with salt and pepper. Roast for about 20 minutes, until fork tender. Set aside.

3. Meanwhile, heat the coconut oil in a large saucepan on a medium heat and soften the onion with a generous pinch of salt. Add the garlic and ginger and cook for 1 minute. Add the spices and cook for a further minute. Add the tomatoes and chilli and cook for 1 more minute.

4. Add the split peas and pour in 750ml of the stock. Simmer for 30 minutes, until tender. Stir occasionally and add more stock if it's all starting to look a little too dry. Taste and season with salt and pepper as needed. When it's cooked, I like to pulse the dahl just a few times with a handheld blender to create some texture.

5. While the dahl is cooking, soft-boil your eggs in a saucepan of water for 6 minutes. Remove from the pan and cool under cold running water to stop them cooking, then halve.

6. Spoon the dahl into bowls, squeeze over the lemon juice, scatter over the coriander leaves and drizzle with chilli oil (if using). Then top with the roasted carrots and halved soft-boiled eggs.

TIP: Soak the split peas overnight to help soften and reduce their cook time (to around 20 minutes) or use red lentils, which cook faster (in around 15 minutes).

Greens and Beans
Taco Salad
(with spiced tofu 'meat')

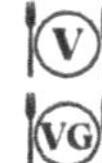
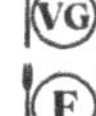

2–3 SERVINGS

Prep time: 15 mins · Cook time: 20 mins

2 generous servings: 31g protein · 14g fibre · 475 cals · 10 plants

3 lighter meals: 21g protein · 9.5g fibre · 318 cals · 10 plants

- » 225g firm tofu (or tempeh), grated
- » 1 tbsp olive oil
- » 1 tsp smoked paprika
- » 1 tsp ground cumin
- » 1 tsp garlic granules
- » Pinch of chilli flakes
- » 1 × 400g tin black beans, drained and rinsed
- » 150g mixed leafy greens (e.g. rocket, watercress and romaine lettuce)
- » 120g shredded red and green cabbage
- » 4 radishes, thinly sliced to serve
- » 1 lime, cut into wedges to serve

For the salsa:
- » 1 small avocado, diced
- » 1 small red onion, finely diced
- » 4 radishes, finely diced
- » 1 large tomato, diced

1. Combine the salsa ingredients in a small bowl and set to one side.
2. In a medium frying pan on a medium heat, fry the grated tofu (or tempeh) with the oil, spices, garlic granules, chilli flakes and some salt and pepper for 10–15 minutes, until it browns and starts to crisp.
3. Add the beans, leafy greens and cabbage and heat through for about 5 minutes.
4. Serve in bowls, topped with the salsa, radishes and lime wedges.

Miso Salmon/ Tofu Plant Bowl

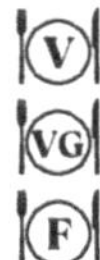

2 SERVINGS

Prep time: 10 mins · Cook time: 20 mins

With salmon: 34g protein · 9g fibre · 550 cals · 7 plants

With tofu: 24g protein · 10g fibre · 400 cals · 8 plants

- » 2 salmon fillets (180g total) or 1 block (225g) firm smoked tofu
- » 120g frozen edamame beans
- » 250g broccoli florets
- » 1 pouch (250g) cooked brown rice
- » 1 red chilli, sliced
- » Handful of coriander leaves
- » 2 tsp sesame seeds

For the miso sauce:
- » 1 tbsp white miso
- » 1 tbsp soy sauce
- » 1 tbsp maple syrup or honey
- » 1 tsp sesame oil
- » 1–2 tbsp warm water to loosen

1. Preheat oven to 200°C (180°C fan)/400°F.
2. In a small bowl mix together all the ingredients for the miso sauce.
3. Place the salmon or tofu in a baking dish and coat with half the miso sauce. Roast the salmon for 10–12 minutes, until it turns opaque and flakes

easily; roast the tofu for 18–20 minutes, until golden on the outside.

4. Meanwhile, cook the edamame beans in a medium saucepan of boiling water for 5 minutes. At the same time, put a colander or metal sieve on top of the saucepan and place the broccoli in it. Put a lid on top and steam the broccoli for about 5 minutes, until just tender.

5. When everything is ready, build your bowls. Top the rice with the broccoli, edamame, salmon or tofu and spoon over the remaining sauce. Finish with chilli, coriander and sesame seeds.

One-Pan Harissa Chicken and Veg

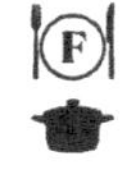

2 SERVINGS

Prep time: 5 mins · Cook time: 30 mins

38g protein · 10g fibre · 540 cals · 8+ plants

» 2 small (120g each) chicken breasts, cut into small bite-sized pieces
» 1 small courgette, cut into chunks
» 1 pepper, cut into chunks
» 1 red onion, cut into wedges
» ½ bulb of fennel, sliced
» 1 small (100g) sweet potato, cut into chunks (skin on if you want extra fibre – just give it a good scrub!)
» 2 tbsp harissa paste
» 1 tbsp olive oil
» 1 pouch (250g) cooked quinoa
» 1 small lemon, halved
» Handful of fresh herbs to serve (I like parsley and basil, but any will do)

1. Preheat oven to 200°C (180°C fan)/400°F.
2. In a roasting tin, toss to coat the chicken and veg in the harissa paste and oil. Roast in the oven for 25–30 minutes, until lightly charred around the edges and cooked all the way through.
3. About 5 minutes before the end of the cooking time, add the quinoa to the tin and mix together

well. Return to the oven for **5** minutes to warm through. Season with salt and pepper to taste.

4. Divide between two bowls. Serve with a squeeze of lemon and the fresh herbs.

Cavolo Nero Anchovy Linguine

4 SERVINGS

Prep time: 10 mins · Cook time: 15 mins

40g protein · 21g fibre · 465 cals · 7 plants

- » 250–300g wholewheat pasta or mung bean fettuccine
- » 150g cavolo nero, stalks removed and roughly chopped
- » 3 tbsp olive oil
- » 30g anchovies from a jar or tin, drained and roughly chopped
- » 3 garlic cloves, minced
- » 100g frozen peas
- » 30g pine nuts
- » Small handful of parsley
- » 3 tbsp nutritional yeast (or 30g Parmesan/ vegetarian hard cheese, grated)
- » Zest of 1 lemon
- » Pinch of chilli flakes to taste

1. Cook the pasta in a large pan of salted boiling water according to the packet instructions.
2. In a wide pan, gently fry the cavolo nero in 1 tbsp of the oil for 3–4 minutes.
3. Add the anchovies and garlic, stir-fry for 1–2 minutes, adding a splash of water when it starts to stick to the pan.

4. Put the frozen peas in a sieve and run under hot water for 20 seconds.

5. Blend the cavolo nero and peas with the pine nuts, parsley, nutritional yeast (or Parmesan/vegetarian hard cheese), the remaining 2 tbsp oil and the lemon zest, to a thick green sauce (loosen with pasta water if needed).

6. Toss the drained hot pasta in the sauce and serve with black pepper and chilli flakes.

Chicken, Chickpea and Feta Tray Bake

4 SERVINGS

Prep time: 10 mins · Cook time: 30 mins

36.5g protein · 11g fibre · 475 cals · 8+ plants

» 1 × 400g tin chickpeas, drained, rinsed and patted dry with paper towel
» 400g chicken breast, diced
» 2 sweet potatoes (about 600g), peeled and diced
» 1 courgette, sliced
» 1 red pepper, sliced
» 1 medium red onion, cut into wedges
» 2 tbsp olive oil
» 1 tsp dried oregano
» 1 tsp smoked paprika
» 2 handfuls of spinach or baby kale
» 100g feta, crumbled
» A few pitted black olives
» Fresh basil, to serve

1. Preheat oven to 230°C (210°C fan)/450°F. Line a roasting tray with baking parchment.
2. Spread the chickpeas, chicken, sweet potatoes, courgette, pepper and red onion on the lined roasting tray. Drizzle with the olive oil, sprinkle with oregano and paprika and season with salt and pepper. Toss well to coat.

3. Roast for 25–30 minutes, turning once halfway through, until the veg is slightly crisp and the chicken is cooked through.
4. Scatter over the spinach (or baby kale) and feta while still warm, letting the spinach wilt slightly. Finish with the olives and fresh basil to serve.

TIP: Swap the chicken for sautéed prawns, seared salmon or crispy tofu cubes.

Harissa Mixed Bean Stew 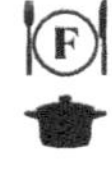

4 SERVINGS

Prep time: 5 mins · Cook time: 20 mins

25g protein · 10g fibre · 413 cals · 7 plants

- » 1 tbsp olive oil
- » 1 medium onion, finely chopped
- » 3 garlic cloves, chopped
- » Pinch of salt
- » 1 tbsp harissa paste (or more for extra heat)
- » 1 x 400g tin chopped tomatoes
- » 500ml vegetable stock
- » 1 × 400g tin borlotti beans, drained and rinsed
- » 1 x 400g tin haricot beans, drained and rinsed
- » Mixed handful of parsley and basil, chopped
- » 150g ricotta (optional)
- » 400g smoked mackerel fillets, flaked
- » 4 slices of sourdough bread

1. Heat the oil in a large saucepan on a low-medium heat and gently cook the onion and garlic with a pinch of salt, until soft.
2. Stir in the harissa paste for 1 minute. Add the tomatoes, stock and beans. Simmer, uncovered, for 12–15 minutes, until thickened. Season well with salt and pepper. Remove from the heat and stir in the herbs.
3. Serve with a spoon of ricotta on top (if using), the flaked mackerel and a slice of sourdough.

TIP: Swap smoked mackerel for tinned for a cheaper option or 300g of crispy tofu for a plant-based option.

CHAPTER 7

Fibre-filled extras

Sometimes it's the little things that make the biggest difference. These extras are the finishing touches that transform an ordinary day into a fibre-packed one – the snacks, sides, toppings and small-but-mighty additions that layer on flavour *and* extra grams of fibre without any extra fuss.

In this section, you'll find everything from Crispy Garlic Beans on p. 204 and Air Fryer Broccoli Fries on p. 202 to Blackberry Chia Jam on p. 210, No-Knead Seed Loaf on p. 205, Red Lentil Wraps on p. 206 and even sweet fibre boosters like Chickpea Blondies on p. 211 and Cookie Dough Energy Balls on p.213. They're quick, adaptable and most have been designed to be made ahead or thrown together on busy days.

Keep a few of these in your fridge or freezer and you'll always have an easy way to turn a simple bowl, salad or tray bake into something more nourishing, more satisfying and naturally richer in fibre. These are the building blocks I rely on in my own kitchen – and you'll soon see how effortlessly they slot into the recipes that follow.

The recipes at a glance

Air Fryer Broccoli Tots

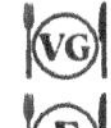

3 SERVINGS

Prep time: 10 mins · Cook time: 15 mins
10g protein · 3g fibre · 160 cals · 3 plants

» 1 medium head of broccoli (around 150g), grated (keep the stalks for my Air fryer broccoli fries on p. 202)
» ½ small red onion, finely chopped
» 1 garlic clove, minced
» 1 egg, lightly whisked
» 50g Cheddar, grated
» 40g breadcrumbs

1. Steam the grated broccoli for 2 minutes, then squeeze out the moisture.
2. In a bowl, mix the broccoli with the onion, garlic, egg, Cheddar and breadcrumbs, and season with salt and pepper. Shape into 12 small tots.
3. Lay them in a single layer in the air fryer and cook at 180°C for 10–12 minutes, shaking halfway, until golden and crisp on the outside.

TIP: If you don't have an air fryer, roast the tots on a baking tray in an oven preheated to 200°C (180°C fan)/400°F for 20 minutes, checking occasionally to make sure they don't burn.

Air Fryer Broccoli Fries

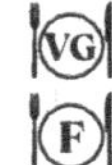

2 SERVINGS

Prep time: 5 mins · Cook time: 10 mins
8g protein · 4g fibre · 140 cals · 2 plants

» Broccoli stalks (around 200g), left over from Air fryer broccoli tots recipe on p. 201, cut into batons
» 1 tsp olive oil
» ½ tsp garlic granules
» 20g finely grated Parmesan/vegetarian hard cheese

1. In a bowl, toss the broccoli stalk batons with the oil, garlic granules and Parmesan/vegetarian hard cheese, and season with salt and pepper.
2. Lay them in a single layer in the air fryer and cook at 180°C for 8–10 minutes, until crisp and lightly browned. Serve as a snack or crunchy side.

TIP: If you don't have an air fryer, roast the fries on a baking tray in an oven preheated to 200°C (180°C fan)/400°F for 20 minutes, checking occasionally to make sure they don't burn.

Roasted Brussels Sprouts with Parmesan

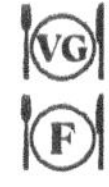

2–3 SERVINGS AS A SIDE

Prep time: 10 minutes · Cook time: 20 minutes

2 servings: 11g protein · 6g fibre · 187 cals · 2 plants

3 servings: 7g protein · 4g fibre · 125 cals · 2 plants

» 300–350g Brussels sprouts, trimmed and halved
» 1 tbsp olive oil
» ½ tsp garlic granules
» 30g Parmesan/vegetarian hard cheese, finely grated

1. Steam the sprouts for 5–6 minutes, until just tender, then drain well. Preheat the oven to 220°C (200°C fan)/425°F.
2. Spread the sprouts on a baking tray lined with baking parchment, then smash them lightly with the bottom of a glass. Toss in the oil, garlic granules and some salt and pepper.
3. Roast for 15–20 minutes, until crisp. Remove from the oven and sprinkle with the Parmesan/vegetarian hard cheese while still hot.

Crispy Garlic Beans

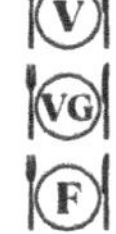

4 SERVINGS

Prep time: 5 mins · Cook time: 20 mins

4g protein · 4g fibre · 88 cals · 2 plants

» 1 x 400g tin cannellini beans, drained, rinsed and patted really dry using paper towel
» 1½ tbsp olive oil
» 1–2 tsp garlic granules

1. Preheat the oven to 180°C (160°C fan)/350°F.
2. Spread out the beans in a roasting tin, drizzle with the oil and season with the garlic granules and salt and pepper. Mix well to combine (I use my hands).
3. Roast in the oven for 15–20 minutes, until crisp and golden (check intermittently to ensure they're not burning). Remove from the oven and allow to cool in the tin slightly before eating.

TIP: Best eaten fresh for crunchiness as a snack or as a topper on soups and salads.

No-Knead Seed Loaf

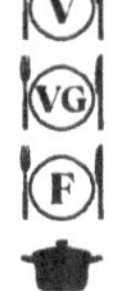

10 SLICES

Prep time: 10 mins · Cook time: 40 mins

10g protein · 9g fibre · 280 cals · 7 plants

- » 130g sunflower seeds
- » 100g ground flaxseeds
- » 50g walnuts, roughly chopped
- » 40g pumpkin seeds
- » 150g rolled oats
- » 2 tbsp chia seeds
- » 4 tbsp psyllium husk
- » 1 tsp fine salt
- » 3 tbsp melted coconut oil or olive oil
- » 350ml water

1. Combine all the dry ingredients in a large mixing bowl. Stir in the melted coconut oil (or olive oil) and water until it forms a thick, uniform batter. Cover and leave to hydrate at room temperature for at least 1 hour or overnight.
2. Preheat the oven to 200°C (180°C fan)/400°F. Line a 900g loaf tin with baking parchment.
3. Press the mixture into the lined loaf tin and bake for 40 minutes, until golden brown on top. Cool fully in the tin, before removing and slicing.

TIP: Because the bread has no preservatives, it won't stay fresh for ages but it freezes well, just remember to slice it first.

Red Lentil Wraps

6 WRAPS

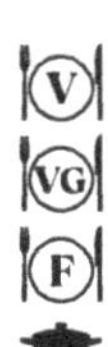

Prep time: 10 mins (+ 3 hours soaking time) ·
Cook time: 15 mins

6.5g protein · 4.5g fibre · 100 cals · 3 plants

» 150g dried red lentils
» 350ml water
» ½ tsp ground cumin (optional)
» ¼ tsp turmeric (optional)
» Pinch of salt
» Olive or avocado oil, for frying

1. Rinse the lentils thoroughly under cold running water. Transfer to a bowl and leave to soak for a minimum of 3 hours in the fridge.
2. Rinse the soaked lentils again under running water and then put in a blender, along with 350ml water, the spices (if using) and a generous pinch of salt. Blitz to a runny, lump-free batter consistency.
3. To cook the wraps, heat a lightly oiled frying pan over a medium-high heat. Add 2–3 tbsp batter per wrap to the hot pan (the mixture should sizzle as it hits the pan), flatten into a circular shape with the back of a spoon or ladle, and cook for 2–3 minutes on each side until golden on both sides. Don't flip too early; wait until the wrap is fully cooked and has turned golden underneath before flipping, otherwise it will probably break. Fill with your favourite

wrap ingredients or serve alongside soups, dahls and stews.

TIP: Keep any leftover cooked wraps in the fridge for up to 4 days. You can briefly reheat them in a lightly oiled hot pan or in the microwave.

Apple and Raspberry Buckwheat Muffins

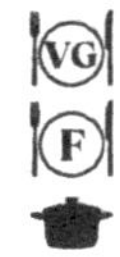

MAKES 10

Prep time: 15 mins · Cook time: 20 mins

5.5g protein · 2g fibre · 165 cals · 8+ plants

» 1 medium apple, chopped into small chunks
» 120g buckwheat flour
» 30g oat bran
» 30g ground flaxseed
» 1 tsp baking powder
» ½ tsp bicarbonate of soda
» 1 tsp ground cinnamon
» 60g light brown sugar
» Pinch of salt
» 30g chopped walnuts
» 30g sunflower seeds
» 1 egg
» 70ml milk (of your choice)
» 30ml olive oil
» 120g yoghurt of choice (I use 0% fat Greek yoghurt)
» ¼ tsp vanilla bean extract (or paste) (optional)
» 20 raspberries

1. Preheat oven to 200°C (180°C fan)/400°F. Line a muffin tray with 10 muffin cases.
2. In a large mixing bowl, combine the chopped apple and all the dry ingredients.

3. In a separate bowl or jug, combine the remaining ingredients, apart from the raspberries.

4. Mix the wet ingredients into the dry ingredients to form a thick batter.

5. Spoon the batter into the 10 muffin cases, pressing 2 raspberries into each one. Bake for 20 minutes, until golden and set. Allow them to cool fully before storing in an airtight container. They will keep for up to 3 days.

Blackberry Chia Jam

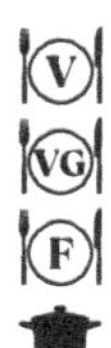

8 X 50G SERVINGS

Prep time: 5 mins · Cook time: 5 mins
1.5g protein · 3g fibre · 30 cals · 2 plants

» 400g blackberries (fresh or frozen)
» 2 tbsp chia seeds
» Juice of 1 lime (or lemon)

1. Place the berries in a small saucepan on a low heat for 5 minutes or so, until they start to soften.
2. Mash them with the back of a fork or potato masher to break them down to a pulp (you can keep them slightly chunkier if you prefer). Remove from the heat and stir in the chia seeds and lime (or lemon) juice.
3. Allow to cool and pour into an airtight container. Store in the fridge for up to a week.

Chickpea Blondies

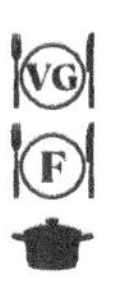

9 SERVINGS

Prep time: 10 mins · Cook time: 25 mins

4.5g protein · 3.5g fibre · 130 cals · 5 plants

- » 1 × 400g tin chickpeas, drained and rinsed
- » 1 medium banana
- » 1 egg or 1 flax egg (1 tbsp ground flaxseeds + 3 tbsp water)
- » 2 tbsp smooth peanut butter
- » 2 tbsp maple syrup or honey
- » ½ tsp vanilla bean extract (or paste)
- » 60g ground oats or ground almonds
- » Pinch of salt
- » 40g dark chocolate chips

1. Preheat oven to 200°C (180°C fan)/400°F and line a 20cm-square tin with baking parchment.
2. Blend the chickpeas, banana, egg (or flax egg), peanut butter, maple syrup (or honey) and vanilla extract in a food processor until smooth. You can combine by hand if you don't have a food processor, the consistency will just be a little chunkier.
3. Fold in the ground oats or almonds, salt and chocolate chips.
4. Spread evenly in the lined tin and bake for 20–25 minutes, until golden at the edges. Cool completely in the tin before slicing into 9 squares; they will firm up as they cool.

Healthier Oat Bran Cookies

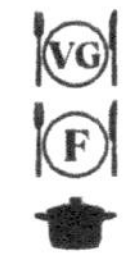

MAKES 8

Prep time: 5 mins · Cook time: 12 mins

4.5g protein · 2.5g fibre · 145 cals · 3+ plants

» 120g oat bran
» 40g ground almonds
» 1 egg, lightly whisked
» 60g maple syrup or honey
» 30g olive oil (though any will do)
» Pinch of salt
» 1 tsp vanilla bean extract (or paste)
» 1 tsp ground cinnamon
» 50g dark chocolate chips

1. Preheat oven to 200°C (180°C fan)/400°F. Line a baking tray with baking parchment.
2. In a large bowl, mix all the ingredients together until well combined.
3. Scoop and shape into 8 balls. Place on the lined baking tray and flatten each ball slightly.
4. Bake for 10–12 minutes, until the edges are golden.

TIP: The cookies will keep in an airtight container for up to 5 days.

Cookie Dough Energy Balls

MAKES 20

Prep time: 20 mins

3g protein · 2g fibre · 85 cals · 5+ plants

» 1 large jar (570g) chickpeas (400g drained weight)
» 40g ground flaxseeds (or ground oats)
» 100g smooth peanut or seed butter (heat briefly in a saucepan if it feels too thick (i.e. it's the slightly harder stuff that you often end up with at the end of the jar)
» 60ml honey or maple syrup
» 60g dark chocolate chips
» 1 tsp ground cinnamon
» 1 tsp vanilla bean extract (or paste)
» Pinch of salt

1. Put the chickpeas in a blender and pulse until really well broken down but not to the point where the mixture becomes too 'wet'. We're looking for a mashed consistency rather than puréed. Alternatively, use a potato masher and mash in a bowl. Fold in the rest of the ingredients and combine well.
2. Roll into 20 balls and store in an airtight container in the fridge – they will keep for at least a week.

TIP: I use jarred chickpeas in this recipe because they're so much bigger and fluffier and so have a better consistency, but the recipe will work just fine with tinned chickpeas.

Air-Popped Popcorn – Sweet and Savoury

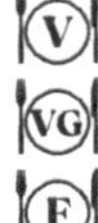

2 SERVINGS

Prep time: 5 mins · Cook time: 5 mins

Sweet base: 3g protein · 5g fibre · 108 cals · 1 plant

Savoury base: 5g protein · 5.5g fibre · 110 cals · 1 plant

» 1 tbsp olive oil (or alternative)
» 60g popping corn kernels

1. Put the oil in a large saucepan with a tight-fitting lid and place on a medium-high heat. When the oil is hot, add 1–2 test kernels to the oil and cover with the lid. Once the test kernels pop, remove from the heat and add the rest of the kernels.
2. Cover the pot again with the lid and carefully shake the pan to cover all the kernels with the oil. Return the pan to the heat and wait to hear the kernels start popping. Shake the pan a few times to prevent burning.
3. When the popping slows down to around 1–2 seconds between pops, remove the pan from the heat, take off the lid (being careful of the trapped steam) and empty the popcorn into a serving bowl.

Maple cinnamon

» 2 tsp maple syrup
» ½–1 tsp ground cinnamon to taste

1. Toss the lightly oiled warm popcorn in the maple syrup and sprinkle with the cinnamon.

Cheesy savoury

» 2 tsp nutritional yeast or finely grated Parmesan/ vegetarian hard cheese

1. Toss the lightly oiled popcorn in the nutritional yeast, Parmesan or vegetarian hard cheese and lightly season with salt.

Pear and Courgette Cake

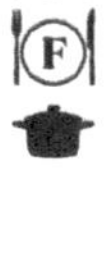

12 SLICES

Prep time: 10 mins · Cook time: 40 mins

4g protein · 3.5g fibre · 200 cals · 7 plants

- » 150g wholemeal spelt flour
- » 50g light brown sugar
- » 50g ground flaxseeds
- » 1 tsp baking powder
- » ½ tsp bicarbonate of soda
- » 1 tsp ground cinnamon
- » ½ tsp ground ginger
- » Pinch of salt
- » 50g pecan nuts, chopped
- » 2 pears, grated
- » 1 small courgette, grated and squeezed
- » 2 eggs, lightly whisked
- » 100ml olive oil (or alternative)

1. Preheat the oven to 190°C (170°C fan)/325°F. Line a 900g loaf tin with baking parchment.
2. In a large bowl, mix together the dry ingredients. In a separate bowl or jug, combine the wet ingredients. Fold the wet ingredients into the dry ingredients to form a thick batter. Tip the batter into the lined loaf tin.
3. Bake for around 40 minutes, until a skewer inserted into the middle comes out clean. Allow to cool in the tin, then remove and cut into slices or squares.

TIP: The cake will keep fresh for 3–4 days in an airtight container.

Pecan Cashew Energy Bombs

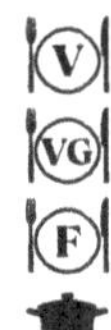

12 SERVINGS

Prep time: 20 mins

3.5g protein · 2.5g fibre · 110 cals · 4 plants

- » 1 x 400g tin chickpeas, drained and rinsed
- » 60g jumbo oats
- » 100g dates, pitted (I like Medjool dates)
- » 60g pecans
- » 60g cashews
- » Pinch of salt
- » 1 tsp vanilla extract

1. In a food processor, pulse all the ingredients into a sticky mass.
2. Roll into 12 balls and store in an airtight container in the fridge – they will keep for at least a week. Alternatively, freeze and take out as needed. Allow to soften for a few minutes before eating.

Raspberry and Pecan Black Bean Brownies

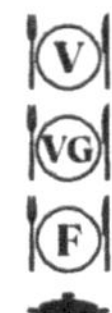

9 SERVINGS

Prep time: 15 mins · Cook time: 20 mins

3.5g protein · 4.5g fibre · 125 cals · 7 plants

» 1 x 400g tin black beans, drained and rinsed
» 2 tbsp cacao powder (or cocoa powder)
» 40g ground flaxseeds
» 60ml maple syrup
» 120ml unsweetened soya milk (or milk of choice)
» 1 tbsp coconut oil
» 100g raspberries
» 50g dark chocolate chips
» 10 pecan halves

1. Preheat oven to 180°C (160°C fan)/350°F. Line a 20cm-square tin with baking parchment.
2. Blend all the ingredients except the raspberries, chocolate chips and pecans in a Nutribullet or high-speed blender until you have a thick but spreadable mixture. You may have to stop and start the blender and scrape down the sides as needed. If it's too thick, add a splash more milk.
3. Fold in the raspberries and half the chocolate chips.
4. Spoon the mixture into the lined tin and smooth over the surface until flat. Scatter the remaining chocolate chips and the pecans on top and bake for 15–20 minutes – the top will be firm to the touch

but inside will still be quite fudgy (it will firm up as it cools).

5. Remove from the oven and allow to cool in the tin. Remove, using the baking parchment as handles, and cut into 9 squares.

TIP: Serve with a generous spoonful of Greek yoghurt (this will bump up the protein, too) and a light dusting of cinnamon.

Summer Fruits with Tahini Sauce

V VG F

2 SERVINGS

Prep time: 15 mins

10.5g protein · 10g fibre · 350 cals · 10+ plants

- » 1 nectarine or peach, stone removed and cut into slices or chunks
- » 100g fresh raspberries
- » 100g fresh blackberries
- » 100g fresh cherries, halved and stones removed
- » 100g pomegranate seeds
- » 2 tbsp mixed seeds to serve

For the tahini sauce:
- » 2 tbsp runny tahini
- » 1 tbsp honey or maple syrup
- » ½ tsp ground cinnamon

1. Arrange the fruit in two serving bowls. Whisk the tahini sauce ingredients together with a tablespoon of water and drizzle over the fruit. Top each bowl with the seeds.

TIP: Serve with a dollop of Greek yoghurt on the side to boost the protein or a splash of kefir for a gut boost.

TIP: You can swap the fruits for whatever is in season.

CHAPTER 8

30g fibre meal plans and shopping lists

Meal plans

Because the majority of us prepare breakfast and lunch for ourselves, but tend to eat more socially in the evening (i.e. with flatmates, partners, family), I've ensured all the meal plans accommodate one person for breakfast and lunch, and two people for dinner. All you need to do is double the quantities if you're cooking dinner for a family of four, or halve them if you're only looking after yourself.

You will notice that meals are often repeated to minimise time spent in the kitchen and to make the most of the batch-friendly recipes. Feel free to make your own meal plan using the empty template at the end of this chapter.

Flexitarian Meal Plan

Day	Breakfast	Lunch	Dinner
Monday	Chia Pudding Three Ways	Chicken, Avocado and Quinoa Nourish Bowl	Chicken, Chickpea and Feta Tray Bake
Tuesday	Chia Pudding Three Ways	Chicken, Avocado and Quinoa Nourish Bowl	Chicken, Chickpea and Feta Tray Bake
Wednesday	Chia Pudding Three Ways	Easy Minestrone Soup	Dahl with Roasted Carrots and Egg
Thursday	Toasted Rye Porridge with Blackberry Chia Jam	Easy Minestrone Soup	Dahl with Roasted Carrots and Egg
Friday	Smashed Peas and Edamame Beans on Rye	Crushed Chickpea-Stuffed Pitta	50:50 Spag Bol
Saturday	Turmeric Kedgeree	One-Pot Creamy White Beans	50:50 Spag Bol
Sunday	Salted Caramel Overnight Oats	One-Pot Creamy White Beans	Cavolo Nero Anchovy Linguine

Shopping List: Flexitarian Plan

Fresh Produce

- Lemons (2–3)
- 1 small avocado
- 8 radishes
- 80g blueberries (fresh or frozen)
- 1 mango
- 3–4 brown onions
- 3 red onions
- 5 carrots
- 3 celery sticks
- 1 leek
- 2 medium courgettes
- 2 red peppers
- 2 sweet potatoes (approx. 600g total)
- 6 medium tomatoes
- Fresh basil (small bunch)
- Fresh parsley (1 small bunch)
- Fresh coriander (1–2 small bunches)
- Fresh mint (1 small bunch)
- Garlic bulbs (2)
- Fresh ginger
- 1 green chilli
- Spinach (1 bag)
- Kale (1 bag)
- Rocket (1 small bag)
- Broccoli sprouts
- Cavolo nero (150g)

Cupboard Staples

- Chickpeas (3 × 400g tins total)
- Cooked lentils (1 × 400g tin)
- Green lentils (1 × 400g tin)
- White beans (2 × 400g tins or 1 × 700g jar)
- Chopped tomatoes (3–4 × 400g)
- Cannellini beans (1 × 400g tin)
- Anchovies (1 small jar or tin)
- Wholegrain or Dijon mustard
- Capers
- Black olives
- Olive oil
- Coconut oil
- Chilli crisp oil
- Maple syrup or honey
- Tomato purée
- Sauerkraut (optional)
- Yellow split peas (250g)
- Brown basmati rice pouch (250g cooked)
- Wholewheat spaghetti (300g)
- Wholewheat pasta or mung bean fettuccine (250–300g)
- Chickpea orzo (250g)
- Jumbo oats
- Rye flakes
- Chia seeds
- Ground flaxseeds
- Pistachios
- Hazelnuts
- Coconut flakes

- Cacao nibs or dark chocolate
- Pine nuts (30g)
- Turmeric
- Ground coriander
- Ground cumin
- Cumin seeds
- Garam masala
- Ground cinnamon
- Smoked paprika
- Sumac
- Dried oregano
- Chilli flakes
- Salt and black pepper
- Vegetable stock
- Nutritional yeast (or swap for Parmesan/ vegetarian hard cheese)

Frozen

- Frozen peas (1 medium bag)
- Soffritto mix (1 bag)
- Frozen edamame beans
- Optional: frozen blueberries (or fresh)
- Optional: frozen mango (or fresh)

Breads & Grains

- Wholemeal pittas (3)
- Seeded sourdough or rye bread
- Wholewheat pasta or spaghetti
- Brown basmati rice pouch (250g cooked)
- Quinoa pouch (250g cooked)

Dairy / Chilled

- Milk of choice (approx. 2 L)
- Yoghurt of choice (approx. 500g)
- Cottage cheese (75g)
- Feta cheese (approx. 115g)
- Parmesan, vegetarian hard cheese or nutritional yeast
- Eggs (6)

Vegetarian Meal Plan

Day	Breakfast	Lunch	Dinner
Monday	Soaked Pearl Barley Porridge with Kiwi	Halloumi Power Bowl with Figs and Honey-Lemon Dressing	Quick Ribollita
Tuesday	Chia Pudding Three Ways	Leek, Broccoli and Potato Soup with Fennel and Miso	Quick Ribollita
Wednesday	Chia Pudding Three Ways	Leek, Broccoli and Potato Soup with Fennel and Miso	Veg-Squeezed Mac and Cheese
Thursday	Cherry Bakewell Overnight Oats	Crispy Chilli Oil Buckwheat Noodles	Veg-Squeezed Mac and Cheese
Friday	Cherry Bakewell Overnight Oats	Coconut Lentils with Crispy Kale	Broccoli Fried Rice with Crispy Egg
Saturday	Maple Pecan Baked Pears	Coconut Lentils with Crispy Kale	Cheesy Green Orzo Bake
Sunday	Shakshuka with Zhoug	Tomato and Red Pepper Pearl Barley Risotto	Cheesy Green Orzo Bake

Shopping List: Vegetarian Plan

Fresh Produce

- Kiwi fruit (2)
- Ripe pears (2)
- Cherries (small punnet or swap for frozen)
- Fresh figs (2)
- Blueberries (small punnet or frozen)
- Lemons (2–3)
- Large leek (2)
- Brown onions (4)
- Peppers (2–3)
- Butternut squash (300g)
- Broccoli (2 medium heads)
- Celery sticks (2)
- Fennel bulb
- Cherry tomatoes (300g)
- Medium tomatoes (7)
- Mixed crunchy veg (approx. 150g – e.g., snap peas, carrot, peppers)
- Curly kale or cavolo nero (approx. 200g)
- Spinach (approx. 3–4 handfuls total)
- Mixed greens or watercress (approx. 80g)
- Fresh coriander (1–2 bunches)
- Fresh mint (1 small bunch)
- Ginger
- Garlic bulb (2)
- Jalapeños or green chillies (2–3)
- Wholemeal pittas (2)
- Large bag mixed salad leaves

Cupboard Staples

- Cannellini beans (2 × 400g tins)
- Haricot beans (1 × 400g tin)
- Chopped tomatoes (1 × 400g tin)
- Full-fat coconut milk (1 × 400ml tin)
- Tomato purée
- Dried red lentils (200g)
- Cooked freekeh or bulgur wheat pouch (250g)
- Olive oil
- Chilli crisp oil
- Soy sauce
- Maple syrup or honey
- Mustard (any type)
- White miso
- Vanilla extract or paste
- Almond extract
- Pecans
- Shelled hemp seeds
- Almonds
- Hazelnuts
- Pistachios
- Mixed seeds
- Pumpkin seeds
- Black sesame seeds
- Breadcrumbs
- Nut or seed butter
- Cacao or cocoa powder
- Ground cinnamon
- Nutmeg
- Ground cumin
- Ground cardamom

- Chilli flakes
- Dried rosemary
- Dried oregano
- Garam masala
- Turmeric
- Mustard seeds
- Cumin seeds
- Salt and pepper

Frozen

- Frozen peas (1 bag)
- Frozen blueberries (or fresh)
- Frozen cherries (or fresh)

Breads & Grains

- Pearl barley
- Jumbo oats
- Wholewheat macaroni or legume pasta (175g)
- Chickpea orzo (250g)
- Buckwheat soba noodles (150g)
- Seeded sourdough loaf
- Wholemeal pittas (2)

Dairy/Chilled

- Milk of choice (2 cartons)
- Yoghurt of choice (approx. 700g total)
- Halloumi (100g)
- Cheddar (approx. 250g total)
- Vegetarian hard cheese (110g total)
- Eggs (6)
- Butter

Vegan Meal Plan

Day	Breakfast	Lunch	Dinner
Monday	Chia Pudding Three Ways	Crushed Chickpea-Stuffed Pitta	Quick Ribollita
Tuesday	Chia Pudding Three Ways	Easy Minestrone Soup	Quick Ribollita
Wednesday	Black Bean and Herb Avocado Toast	Easy Minestrone Soup	Borlotti Bean Ragú
Thursday	Cherry Bakewell Overnight Oats	Pesto Orzo Salad	Borlotti Bean Ragú
Friday	Cherry Bakewell Overnight Oats	Pesto Orzo Salad	Black Bean Burger
Saturday	Miso Mushrooms on Rye	Raw Pad Thai	Harissa Mixed Bean Stew
Sunday	Soaked Pearl Barley Porridge with Kiwi	One-Pot Creamy White Beans	Harissa Mixed Bean Stew

Shopping List: Vegan Plan

Fresh Produce

- Bananas (2–3)
- Kiwi fruit (2)
- Mushrooms (400g)
- Spring onions (2)
- Parsley (2 small bunches)
- Chives (small bunch)
- Basil (2 small bunches)
- Coriander (2 small bunches)
- Avocados (3–4 total)
- Lemons/limes (6–8 total)
- Red onions (3–4)
- Carrots (6–7 medium)
- Celery sticks (5–6)
- Courgette (1 large)
- Leek (1)
- Tomatoes (4)
- Cherry tomatoes (120g)
- Garlic bulb (1)
- Mixed leafy greens/rocket (large bag or 2–3 small bags)
- Beansprouts (1 large handful)
- Mixed veg for pad Thai (350g)
- Red chilli (1)
- Spinach (large handful)
- Cavolo nero (200g)
- 200g mushrooms (any kind)
- Fresh herbs: dill (small bunch), parsley/basil (large bunch)

- Kiwi fruit (2)
- Mixed salad leaves (1–2 bags)
- Peppers, sugar snaps, mange tout (for Raw pad Thai)
- Cucumber (1)

Frozen

- Peas (1 bag)
- Frozen cherries (1 bag)
- Frozen mixed berries (1 bag)
- Frozen soffritto mix (1 bag)

Cupboard Staples

- Jumbo oats
- Wheat bran
- Ground almonds
- Flaked almonds
- Walnuts
- Pine nuts
- Nut or seed butter
- Pumpkin seeds
- Chia seeds
- Flaxseeds
- Maple syrup
- Vanilla extract/paste
- Almond extract
- Ground cinnamon
- Cacao or cocoa powder
- Coconut flakes
- Olive oil

- Dijon or wholegrain mustard
- Capers
- Sumac
- Chickpeas (3 × 400g tins)
- Black beans (2 × 400g tins)
- Cannellini beans (1 x 400g tin)
- Haricot beans (2 x 400g tins)
- Borlotti beans (2 x 400g tins)
- Chopped tomatoes (6 × 400g tins)
- Tomato purée
- Vegetable stock (cubes or liquid; several litres)
- Dried orzo (200g)
- Wholewheat pasta (150g)
- Mung bean tagliatelle or other pasta (200g)
- Quinoa
- Panko breadcrumbs
- Soy sauce
- Sesame oil
- BBQ sauce
- Harissa paste
- Dried oregano
- Dried rosemary
- Mixed dried herbs
- Garlic granules
- Smoked paprika
- Ground cumin
- Chilli flakes
- Salt and pepper

Plant-Based Dairy Alternatives

- Unsweetened soya milk (large carton)
- Unsweetened soya yoghurt (big tub)
- Coconut milk (1 × 400ml tin)
- Nutritional yeast (large tub; several tbsp required)

Breads/Grains

- Rye bread
- Seeded sourdough
- Wholemeal pittas

Blank meal plan

Day	Breakfast	Lunch	Dinner
Monday			
Tuesday			
Wednesday			
Thursday			
Friday			
Saturday			
Sunday			

Part Three

Your Fibre Toolkit

Fibre Cheat Sheet: Quantities at a Glance

Food	Fibre (g/100g)	Fibre (g/80g portion)
Vegetables		
Avocado (raw)	6.7	5.4
Artichoke (raw)	5.4	4.3
Broad beans (raw)	5.4	4.3
Green peas (raw)	5.1	4.1
Parsnip (raw)	4.9	3.9
Collard greens (raw)	4.0	3.2
Brussels sprouts (raw)	3.8	3.0
Kale (raw)	3.6	2.9
Kohlrabi (raw)	3.6	2.9
Green beans (raw)	3.4	2.7
Fennel (raw)	3.1	2.5
Savoy cabbage (raw)	3.1	2.5
Aubergine (raw)	3.0	2.4
Sweet potato (raw)	3.0	2.4
Carrots (raw)	2.8	2.2
Beetroot (raw)	2.8	2.2
Sweetcorn (raw)	2.7	2.2
Broccoli (raw)	2.6	2.1
Spring onions (raw)	2.6	2.1
Sugar snap peas (raw)	2.6	2.1
Mange tout (raw)	2.6	2.1
Spinach (raw)	2.2	1.8
Potato, baked flesh + skin (raw weight)	2.2	1.8
Red cabbage (raw)	2.1	1.7
Asparagus (raw)	2.1	1.7
Garlic (raw)	2.1	1.7
Butternut squash (raw)	2.0	1.6
Cauliflower (raw)	2.0	1.6

Food	Fibre (g/100g)	Fibre (g/80g portion)
Alfalfa sprouts (raw)	1.9	1.5
Beansprouts (raw)	1.8	1.4
Leeks (raw)	1.8	1.4
Peppers (raw)	1.7	1.4
Red onion (raw)	1.7	1.4
Swiss chard (raw)	1.6	1.3
Rocket (raw)	1.6	1.3
Celery (raw)	1.6	1.3
Tomatoes (raw)	1.2	1.0
Lettuce (raw)	1.2	1.0
Courgette (raw)	1.1	0.9
Mushrooms (raw)	1.0	0.8
Pumpkin (raw)	0.5	0.4
Cucumber (raw)	0.5	0.4
Fruit		
Passion fruit	10.4	8.3
Prunes (dried)	7.1	5.7
Medjool dates	6.7	5.4
Raspberries	6.5	5.2
Guava	5.4	4.3
Blackberries	5.3	4.2
Pomegranate	4.0	3.2
Pear	3.1	2.5
Kiwi fruit	3.0	2.4
Figs (fresh)	2.9	2.3
Banana	2.6	2.1
Blueberries	2.4	1.9
Apple	2.4	1.9
Orange	2.4	1.9
Cherries	2.1	1.7
Strawberries	2.0	1.6

Food	Fibre (g/100g)	Fibre (g/80g portion)
Apricots	2.0	1.6
Rhubarb	1.8	1.4
Tangerines	1.8	1.4
Papaya	1.7	1.4
Nectarines	1.7	1.4
Mango	1.6	1.3
Grapefruit	1.6	1.3
Peaches	1.5	1.2
Pineapple	1.4	1.1
Plums	1.4	1.1
Honeydew melon	0.8	0.6
Watermelon	0.4	0.3
Beans and Legumes		
Psyllium husks	78.0	62.4
Cannellini beans (cooked)	11.3	9.0
Red lentils (dried)	10.8	8.6
Black beans (cooked)	8.7	7.0
Split peas (cooked)	8.3	6.6
Butter beans (cooked)	7.9	6.3
Lentils (green, cooked)	7.8	6.2
Mung beans (cooked)	7.6	6.1
Chickpeas (cooked)	7.6	6.1
Adzuki beans (cooked)	7.3	5.8
Haricot beans (cooked)	7.3	5.8
Puy lentils (cooked)	7.0	5.6
Kidney beans (cooked)	6.4	5.1
Hummus	6.0	4.8
Pinto beans (cooked)	5.5	4.4
Broad beans (cooked)	5.4	4.3
Miso	5.4	4.3
Edamame beans (cooked)	5.2	4.2
Chestnuts	3.0	0.9

Food	Fibre (g/100g)	Fibre (g/30g portion)
Nuts		
Almonds	12.5	3.8
Pistachios	10.6	3.2
Hazelnuts	9.7	2.9
Pecans	9.6	2.9
Macadamias	8.6	2.6
Peanuts	8.0	2.4
Brazil nuts	7.5	2.2
Walnuts	6.7	2.0
Pine nuts	3.7	1.1
Cashews	3.3	1.0

Food	Fibre (g/100g)	Fibre (g/15g portion)
Seeds		
Chia seeds	34.4	5.0
Raw cacao (powder)	33.0	5.0
Ground flaxseed	28.8	4.0
Flaxseeds (whole)	27.3	4.0
Pumpkin seeds	18.4	3.0
Desiccated coconut	16.3	2.0
Sesame seeds	11.8	2.0
Sunflower seeds	11.1	2.0
Tahini	9.3	1.0
Coconut (fresh)	9.0	1.0
Almond butter	6.8	1.0
Peanut butter	6.0	1.0
Cashew butter	3.0	0.5

Food	Fibre (g/100g)	Fibre (g/40g portion)
Grains		
Wheat bran	42.8	17.1
Pearl barley	17.3	6.9
Oat bran	15.4	6.2

Food	Fibre (g/100g)	Fibre (g/40g portion)
Edamame pasta	15.0	6.0
Popcorn	14.5	5.8
Rye crackers	14.0	5.6
Freekeh	12.7	5.1
Bulgur wheat	12.5	5.0
Wholemeal flour	11.2	4.5
Chickpea flour	11.2	4.5
Yellow pea pasta	11.0	4.4
Spelt (whole)	10.7	4.3
Oats	10.6	4.2
Rye flakes	10.1	4.0
Barley flakes	10.1	4.0
Buckwheat flour	10.0	4.0
Wholewheat pasta	8.0	3.2
Wholemeal wrap	7.5	3.0
Wholewheat couscous	7.0	2.8
Quinoa	7.0	2.8
Wholewheat pitta bread	7.0	2.8
Pumpernickel bread	6.5	2.6
Seeded sourdough	6.5	2.6
Wild rice	6.2	2.5
Wholemeal bread	6.0	2.4
Wholewheat noodles	6.0	2.4
Rye bread	5.8	2.3
Couscous	5.0	2.0
Red rice	4.9	2.0
Brown rice	3.5	1.4
Egg noodles	3.2	1.3
White pasta	3.2	1.3
Plain flour	3.0	1.2
Buckwheat soba noodles	3.0	1.2
White bread	2.7	1.1
Basmati rice	2.4	1.0

Plant Diversity Wheel

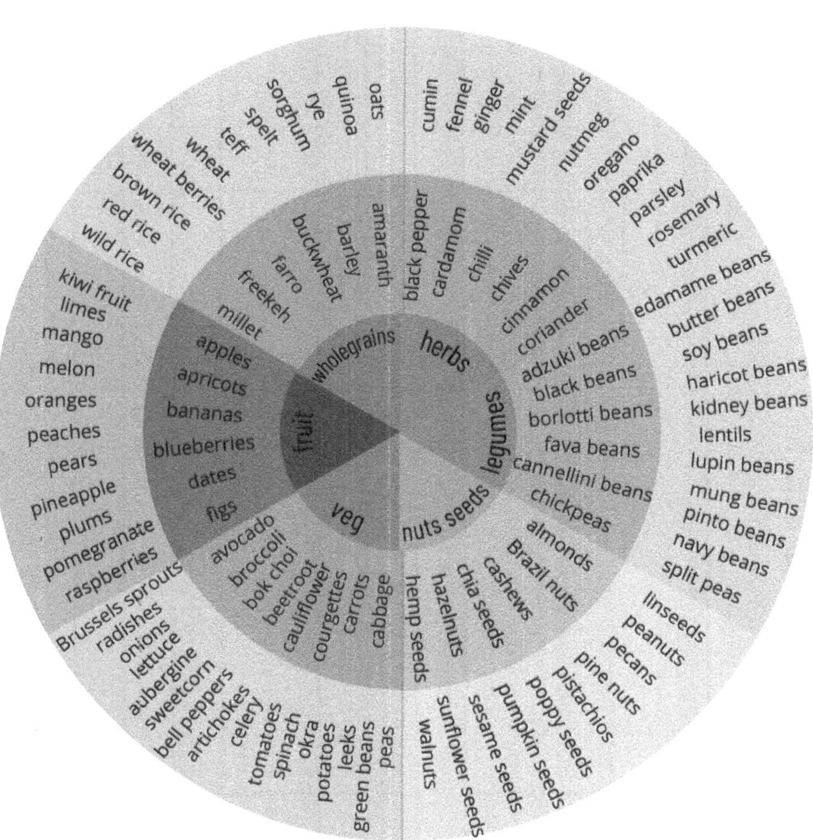

30 Plant Points Tracker

Weekly Plant Tracker

Aim for 30+ plant-based foods per week

VEGETABLES	FRUITS	NUTS & SEEDS	GRAINS	LEGUMES	HERBS & SPICES
Total:	Total:	Total:	Total:	Total:	Total:

Grand Total: /30

References

Chapter 1

1. **Reynolds, A.N. et al. (2019)** 'Carbohydrate quality and human health: a series of systematic reviews and meta-analyses', *The Lancet*, 393(10170), pp. 434–445. **– Higher fibre intakes reduce risk of CVD, type 2 diabetes, colorectal cancer and all-cause mortality and improve weight, blood lipids and glycaemic control.**
2. **Gill, S.K., Rossi, M., Bajka, B. and Whelan, K. (2021)** 'Dietary fibre in gastrointestinal health and disease', *Nature Reviews Gastroenterology & Hepatology*, 18, pp. 101–116. **– Mechanisms by which fibre affects gut motility, microbiota, SCFAs, immunity, bowel function and GI disorders.**
3. **Scientific Advisory Committee on Nutrition (SACN) (2015)** *Carbohydrates and Health.* London: Public Health England. **– UK recommendation of 30g/day fibre for adults, based on systematic review of fibre and chronic disease risk.**
4. **Public Health England (2020)** *National Diet and Nutrition Survey: results from Years 9 to 11 (2016/2017 to 2018/2019).* London: PHE. **– Mean adult fibre intake ~18–19g/day and the vast majority (≈90–95%) fail to reach 30g; also highlights child fibre shortfalls.**
5. **Koh, A. et al. (2016)** 'From dietary fibre to host physiology: short-chain fatty acids as key bacterial metabolites', *Cell*, 165(6), pp. 1332–1345. **– Mechanistic review on fermentation of fibre to SCFAs and their roles in energy metabolism, gut barrier integrity, immunity and hormone signalling.**
6. **Canfora, E.E., Jocken, J.W. and Blaak, E.E. (2015)** 'Short-chain fatty acids in control of body weight and insulin sensitivity', *Nature Reviews Endocrinology*, 11(10), pp. 577–591. **– SCFAs, GLP-1, PYY, appetite regulation, metabolic health and weight.**

7. Brown, L. et al. (1999) 'Cholesterol-lowering effects of dietary fibre: a meta-analysis', *American Journal of Clinical Nutrition*, 69(1), pp. 30–42. – **Soluble/viscous fibre lowers LDL cholesterol.**

8. Whitehead, A., Beck, E.J., Tosh, S. and Wolever, T.M.S. (2014) 'Cholesterol-lowering effects of oat *ß*-glucan: a meta-analysis of randomised controlled trials', *American Journal of Clinical Nutrition*, 100(6), pp. 1413–1421. – **3g/day *ß*-glucans/oats, barley and impact on LDL.**

9. Threapleton, D.E. et al. (2013) 'Dietary fibre intake and risk of cardiovascular disease: systematic review and meta-analysis', *BMJ*, 347, f6879. – **Dose-response relationship between fibre intake and lower CVD risk.**

10. Yao, B. et al. (2014) 'Dietary fibre intake and risk of type 2 diabetes: a dose–response analysis of prospective studies', *European Journal of Epidemiology*, 29, pp. 79–88. – **Higher total and cereal fibre associated with reduced type 2 diabetes risk.**

11. Aune, D. et al. (2011) 'Dietary fibre, whole grains, and risk of colorectal cancer: systematic review and dose-response meta-analysis of prospective studies', *BMJ*, 343, d6617. – **Imperial-led analysis (~2 million participants) showing each additional 10 g/day of fibre associated with ≈10% lower colorectal cancer risk.**

12. Kim, Y. and Je, Y. (2014) 'Dietary fibre intake and total mortality: a meta-analysis of prospective cohort studies', *American Journal of Epidemiology*, 180(6), pp. 565–573. – **Extra 10g/day of fibre linked with ≈10% lower all-cause mortality.**

13. David, L.A. et al. (2014) 'Diet rapidly and reproducibly alters the human gut microbiome', *Nature*, 505(7484), pp. 559–563. – **Gut microbiota composition shift within 24–48 hours of major dietary changes.**

14. Desai, M.S. et al. (2016) 'A dietary fiber-deprived gut microbiota degrades the colonic mucus barrier and enhances pathogen susceptibility', *Cell*, 167(5), pp. 1339–1353.e21. – **Shows low-fibre diets drive microbes to erode the mucous layer, weakening the gut barrier and increasing inflammation and infection risk.**

15. Bowe, W.P. and Logan, A.C. (2011) 'Acne vulgaris, probiotics and the gut–brain–skin axis – back to the future?', *Gut Pathogens*, 3(1), p. 1. – **Link between gut microbiota, systemic inflammation and skin conditions (acne/eczema, etc).**

16. Thorburn, A.N., Macia, L. and Mackay, C.R. (2014) 'Diet,

metabolites, and "western-lifestyle" inflammatory diseases', *Immunity*, 40(6), pp. 833–842. – **SCFAs, immune regulation, allergy/ autoimmunity and the protective role of fibre.**

17. **Camilleri, M. (2019)** 'Leaky gut: mechanisms, measurement and clinical implications in humans', *Gut*, 68(8), pp. 1516–1526. – **Authoritative review on intestinal permeability and factors that influence it, including diet and SCFAs.**

18. **Jacka, F.N. et al. (2017)** 'A randomised controlled trial of dietary improvement for adults with major depression (the "SMILES" trial)'. *BMC Medicine*, 15, p. 23. – **Mediterranean-style, fibre-rich diet significantly improved depression scores vs control.**

19. **Thursby, E. and Juge, N. (2017)** 'Introduction to the human gut microbiota', *Biochemical Journal*, 474(11), pp. 1823–1836. – **Microbiome composition, functions and host interactions.**

20. **Gibson, G.R. et al. (2017)** 'Expert consensus document: The International Scientific Association for Probiotics and Prebiotics (ISAPP) consensus statement on the definition and scope of prebiotics', *Nature Reviews Gastroenterology & Hepatology*, 14(8), pp. 491–502. – **Prebiotics: inulin, FOS, GOS, polyphenols, omega-3.**

21. **Aguilar-Toalá, J.E. et al. (2021)** 'Postbiotics: an evolving term within the functional foods field', *Trends in Food Science & Technology*, 108, pp. 11–26. – **Evidence and consensus around the health effects of postbiotics and fermented foods.**

22. **McDonald, D. et al. (2018)** 'American Gut: an open platform for citizen science microbiome research', *mSystems*, 3(3), e00031-18. – **Individuals eating ≥30 different plant types/week had more diverse gut microbiotas than those eating fewer plants.**

23. **Schnorr, S.L. et al. (2014)** 'Gut microbiome of the Hadza hunter-gatherers', *Nature Communications*, 5, 3654. – **Hadza microbiome diversity linked to high-fibre, plant-rich diets.**

24. **Smits, S.A. et al. (2017)** 'Seasonal cycling in the gut microbiome of the Hadza hunter-gatherers of Tanzania', *Science*, 357(6353), pp. 802–806. – **Evidence on Hadza diet and gut microbial diversity.**

25. **De Filippo, C. et al. (2010)** 'Impact of diet in shaping gut microbiota revealed by a comparative study in children from Europe and rural Africa', *Proceedings of the National Academy of Sciences*, 107(33), pp. 14691–14696. – **Higher-fibre traditional diets associated with more diverse, SCFA-producing microbiota than Western low-fibre diets.**

26. **De Palma, G. et al. (2009)** 'Influence of a gluten-free diet on gut microbiota composition in healthy adult humans', *British*

Journal of Nutrition, 102(8), pp. 1154–1160. **– Gluten-free diet (in non-coeliac adults) reduced Bifidobacterium and Lactobacillus and overall microbial diversity.**

27. **Bharucha, A.E. and Lacy, B.E. (2020)** 'Mechanisms, evaluation, and management of chronic constipation', *Gastroenterology*, 158(5), pp. 1232–1249.e3. **– Higher prevalence of constipation in women and the influence of hormones, pelvic floor and colonic transit.**

28. **Chumpitazi, B.P. and Shulman, R.J. (2016)** 'Dietary carbohydrates and childhood functional gastrointestinal disorders', *Annals of Nutrition & Metabolism*, 68(Suppl. 1), pp. 8–17. **– Importance of fibre and plant foods in paediatric gut health.**

29. **NHS (2021)** *How much fibre do I need?* Available at: NHS.uk (accessed [date]). **– UK fibre targets for adults and children (e.g. ~15g/day for 2–5 year-olds; ~25g for older children/teens).**

30. **Park, Y. et al. (2011)** 'Dietary fibre intake and mortality in the NIH-AARP Diet and Health Study', *Archives of Internal Medicine*, 171(12), pp. 1061–1068. **– Large US cohort study showing higher fibre intake associated with lower total mortality.**

Chapter 2

1. **Whitehead, A., Beck, E. J., Tosh, S. Wolever, T. M. S. (2014).** Cholesterol-lowering effects of oat ß-glucan: A meta-analysis of randomized controlled trials. *American Journal of Clinical Nutrition*, 100(6), 1413–1421. **– Meta-analysis of 28 RCTs confirming that ≥3g/day oat beta-glucan significantly lowers LDL cholesterol.**

2. **Bazzano, L. A., Thompson, A. M., Tees, M. T., Nguyen, C. H., Winham, D. M. (2011).** Non-soy legume consumption lowers cholesterol: A systematic review and meta-analysis. *Nutrition, Metabolism & Cardiovascular Diseases*, 21(2), 94–103. **– Regular consumption of legumes improves cholesterol and stabilises post-meal blood glucose.**

3. **Ulbricht, C., Chao, W., Windsor, R. C., et al. (2009).** Chia seed (Salvia hispanica): An evidence-based systematic review. *Journal of Alternative and Complementary Medicine*, 15(11), 1177–1181. **– Chia seeds provide significant soluble fibre, improves satiety and supports glycaemic control.**

4. **Pan, A., Yu, D., Demark-Wahnefried, W., Franco, O. H., Lin, X. (2009).** Meta-analysis of flaxseed and lignans on blood lipids. *American Journal of Clinical Nutrition*, 90(2), 288–297. **– Flaxseed intake significantly reduces LDL cholesterol and improves digestive regularity.**

5. **Mikkelsen, P. B., Toubro, S., Astrup, A. (2000).** Effect of fat-reduced diets on 24-h energy expenditure: Effects of pectin supplementation. *International Journal of Obesity*, 24, 488–496. – **Pectin slows gastric emptying and post-meal rises in blood sugar.**

6. **Gearry, R., Fukudo, S., Barbara, G., Imaeda, H., Wu, J., et al. (2023).** Consumption of 2 green kiwifruits daily improves constipation and abdominal comfort: Results of an international multicenter randomized controlled trial. *American Journal of Gastroenterology*, 118(6), 1058–1068. – **Two green kiwi fruits per day significantly improve bowel frequency, stool form and abdominal comfort.**

7. **Miller, M. G., Shukitt-Hale, B. (2012).** Berry fruit enhances beneficial signaling in the brain. *Journal of Agricultural and Food Chemistry*, 60(23), 5695–5701. – **Berries' anthocyanins support cognitive function and reduce inflammation.**

8. **Myzak, M. C., Hardin, K., Wang, R., et al. (2006).** Sulforaphane inhibits histone deacetylase activity in vivo and suppresses tumor growth. *Proceedings of the National Academy of Sciences*, 103(33), 12541–12546. – **Sulforaphane's potent antioxidant and cellular-protective effects.**

9. **Nilsson, A. C., Ostman, E. M., Holst, J. J., Björck, I. M. (2008).** Including fermented or non-fermented legumes in a meal reduces glucose response and increases satiety. *European Journal of Clinical Nutrition*, 62, 87–95. – **Legumes increase GLP-1 and PYY, contributing to improved satiety and blood sugar stability.**

10. **Ha, V., Sievenpiper, J. L., et al. (2014).** Effect of dietary pulse intake on established therapeutic lipid targets: A systematic review and meta-analysis. *Canadian Medical Association Journal*, 186(8), E252–E262. – **Daily intake of beans/legumes improves LDL cholesterol and cardiometabolic markers.**

11. **Kim, Y., Keogh, J. B., Clifton, P. M. (2017).** Benefits of nuts in the prevention and management of type 2 diabetes. *Nutrients*, 9(11), 1271. – **Nuts improve glycaemic control, satiety, and cardiometabolic health.**

12. **Venn, B. J., Mann J. I. (2004).** Cereal grains, legumes and diabetes. *European Journal of Clinical Nutrition*, 58(11), 1443–1461. – **Lentils significantly reduce post-meal blood glucose responses and improve metabolic markers.**

13. **Aune, D., Keum, N., Giovannucci, E., et al. (2016).** Whole grain consumption and risk of cardiovascular disease, cancer and mortality: Systematic review and dose-response meta-analysis. *BMJ*, 353, i2716. – **Large meta-analysis showing higher wholegrain intake reduces risk of cardiovascular disease and mortality.**

14. **Roberfroid, M. B. (2007).** Inulin-type fructans: Functional food ingredients. *Journal of Nutrition*, 137(11), 2493S–2502S. – **Inulin and fructans in alliums are powerful prebiotics.**

15. **Morris, M. C., Tangney, C. C., Wang, Y., et al. (2018).** Nutrients and bioactives in green leafy vegetables and cognitive decline. *Neurology*, 90(3), e214–e222. – **Higher intakes of leafy greens are linked to slower cognitive decline.**

16. **Kim, Y., Keogh, J. B., Clifton, P. M. (2016).** Polyphenols and health: Gut microbiota and beyond. *Nutrients*, 8(12), 697. – **Cocoa polyphenols influence gut bacteria and metabolic health.**

17. **Navarro, A. M., Martinez-Gonzalez, M. A., et al. (2015).** Coffee consumption and total dietary fibre intake: The SUN cohort study. *Public Health Nutrition*, 18(3), 527–534. – **Brewed coffee contributes measurable soluble fibre to total intake.**

18. **Lampi, A. M., et al. (2013).** Inulin-rich vegetables and health. *Comprehensive Reviews in Food Science and Food Safety*, 12(6), 558–567. – **Artichokes contain some of the highest natural levels of inulin, supporting gut microbial growth.**

19. **Wasser, S. P. (2002).** Medicinal mushrooms as a source of polysaccharides with therapeutic potential. *Applied Microbiology & Biotechnology*, 60, 258–274. – **Mushrooms beta-glucan content and their biological effects.**

20. **Ellett, D. L., et al. (2021).** Psyllium fiber improves lipid and glucose metabolism: A meta-analysis of RCTs. *American Journal of Clinical Nutrition*, 113(2), 327–337. – **Psyllium improves bowel regularity, lowers LDL and supports glycaemic control.**

21. **Fukudo, S., et al. (2021).** Partially hydrolysed guar gum in IBS: Systematic review. *Journal of Gastroenterology and Hepatology*, 36(1), 41–50. – **PHGG improves stool form and reduces IBS symptoms.**

22. **Didari, T., Mozaffari, S., Nikfar, S., Abdollahi, M. (2015).** Probiotics in irritable bowel syndrome: A systematic review and meta-analysis. *World Journal of Gastroenterology*, 21(10), 3072–3084. – **Benefits of specific probiotic strains for IBS symptoms, with strain-specific effects.**

Acknowledgements

My deepest thanks to **Laura Bayliss** for your amazing editorial skills and unwavering patience (not to mention all the poo chat) – it was a tough gig and time was not on our side, but we bloody well did it – I truly couldn't have managed this without you.

Endlessly grateful to you, **Alicja Sieronski** for testing, advising (and much more) on so many of the recipes in this book – your skill, taste buds and insight made everything taste next level. To **Kimberly Espinel**, thank you for the incredible press photos that bring these dishes to life so beautifully, you are just brilliant at what you do. Shout out to you, **Jo Meadows**, for your wise eyes, meticulous proofreading and generous nutrition insights – your invaluable input helped me sleep better at night.

Thank you to **Sam Jackson, Céline Nyssens, Aisling O'Toole, Jasleen Dhindsa**, and the exceptional team working behind the scenes at **Vermilion** for seeing the beauty in fibre, championing the book and guiding it into the world. To my agent, **Valeria Huerta**, this is our third book together, can you believe it?! Thanks for constantly checking in on me and encouraging me from afar.

To **my family**, appreciate you eating ALL THE BEANS – on repeat – and not moaning (too much).

Your gut microbes are quietly (well … not always) thanking you for handling everything I chuck at you.

But most of all, a gigantic thank you to **you** – my readers and followers – for constantly believing in me, cooking along with me and sharing my enthusiasm for no-nonsense nutrition. Your support is the reason this book exists and I am so grateful to be on this journey with you.

@emma.bardwell
www.emmabardwell.com

Index

Note: pages numbers in **bold** refer to diagrams, pages numbers in *italics* refer to information contained in tables.

digestion 13, 19, 29, 34, 60, 66,
  69, 72
digestive aids 111
dinners 44, 58, 98–9, 167–98,
  222
dopamine 23
dressings 164–5; herb 144–5;
  honey-lemon 149; satay 166
drinks 10, 59, 104
dysbiosis 32

'eating the rainbow' 47, *48, 100*
eczema 21, 33
edamame beans 71–2, 94–5,
  131, 190–1; smashed peas and
  edamame beans on rye 130
eggs 131, 138–9; broccoli fried
  rice with crispy egg 172–3;
  dahl with roasted carrots and
  egg 186–7
endometriosis 7, 24
energy balls, cookie dough 213
energy bombs, pecan cashew 217
energy levels 4–5, 18–19, 33–4,
  69, 119; mid-day slumps/
  crashes 11, 18
estrobolome 24–5
excretion 6, 19, 25

Faecalibacterium 36
fats, healthy 112
fennel 105, 152–3, 192–3
fermentation 32, 35, 53, 75, 85,
  104, 106
fermented foods 11, 39, 41, 113,
  115
feta: chicken, chickpea and feta
  tray bake 196–7; whipped feta
  176–7
fibre 1–2; 30:30 rule 46–9;
  abundance 1, 2–3; adding
  an extra 10g a day 45–6;

affordability 2–3; building
up your intake 34, 45–6, 57,
65, 87, 89, 104; children and
57–8, *57;* definition 27–8,
60; and drinks 59; and energy
levels 4, 5, 18–19; FAQs 54–
60; fibre content of common
foods *238–42;* functions of 1,
4–7, 17–25; insoluble 29–30,
61, 65–6, 68–70, 73–5, 80–1,
104; instant wins of 3–4; intake
requirements 42–9, 55–7,
60, *102*, 141; and long-term
health 3–4, 25; magic of eating
more 17–61; overconsumption
57; power of 1, 13; recipes
116, 117–220; shortages 26;
sources of 2, 27–8, 55, 61,
63–79; as superfood 1, 2–4;
supplements 55, 84–7; tracking
the amount you eat 47–9, 59,
243, 244; types of 28–31, *31,*
61; variety/diversity of 42–3;
what counts as fibre 28–31, *31;*
see also soluble fibre
fibre challenge, 10-day 100–1,
  100–1
fibre co-stars 79–84
fibre effect timeline 4–7
fibre hacks 111–16
fibre heroes 61, 63–79
fibre swaps 97–9
fibre toolkit 14, 237, *238–42,*
  243, *244*
fibre-fit quiz 8–12
fibre-friendly life 89–116
fibre-stacking 101–2, *102–3*
figs 149
fish 131, 190–1, 194–5, 198
flavanols *48*
flavones *48*
flavonoids *48*

parsley 126, 160–1, 164–5
partially hydrolysed guar gum (PHGG) 86
pasta 30, 76, 95, 98, 150–1; 50:50 spag bol 174–5; borlotti bean ragú 180–1; cavolo nero anchovy linguine 194–5; legume-based 45, 49, 95, *101*; mac and cheese 182–4; *see also* orzo
peanut butter 211, 213
peanuts 166
pearl barley 29, 76, 99, 115; soaked pearl barley porridge with kiwi 122–3; tomato and red pepper pearl barley risotto 158–9
pears: maple pecan baked pears 132–3; pear and courgette cake 216
peas 37, 71–2, 94, 131, 150–3, 185, 194–5; pea and mint soup 156–7; smashed peas and edamame beans on rye 130
pecan nuts 74, 216; maple pecan baked pears 132–3; pecan cashew energy bombs 217; raspberry and pecan black bean brownies 218–19
pectin *31*, 69, 73
pelvic floor muscles 60
peppermint oil 105
peppers (bell) 138–9, 148, 158–9, 166, 172–3, 192–3, 196–7
perimenopause 68
periods 24, 60, 84
peristalsis 19
pesto: pesto orzo salad 155; pesto toast 154
phenolic acids *48*
physical exercise 105

phytates 55
pine nuts 155, 194–5
pitta, chickpea-stuffed 143
plant-foods: plant diversity wheel **243**; plant point system 47, 49; plant tracker template 48; protein 94; variety of 10, 47–9, 56; weekly plant tracker **244**
plastics, microplastics 6, 19
polycystic ovary syndrome (PCOS) 7, 24
polyphenols 39, 47, 49, 63–4, 67, 72, 113
pomegranate seeds 160–1, 220
poo 13, 49–53; abnormal 52; appearance 9, 49, 50, **51**, 52; bulkers 19, 65; and hormone excretion 24; softeners 19; *see also* bowel movements
popcorn 81–2; air-popped 214–15
porridge: pearl barley 122–3; toasted rye 134–5
postbiotics 37, 41, *42*
potatoes 30, 38; leek, broccoli and potato soup 152–3
power bowl, halloumi 149
prebiotic fibre 30, *31*, 32, 37–41, *42*, 47, 61, 63, 73, 77, 81, 85; custom blends 86; *see also* inulin; polyphenols
pressure cookers 105, 108
probiotics 37, 39–40, *42*, 64, 87–8
progesterone 24, 51, 60
propionate 35, 36, 41
protein 13–14, 56, 67, 72, 74, 84, 94
psyllium 55, 84–5, *100*, 127, 205
pulses 10–11
pumpkin seeds 74, 170–1, 205
PYY 20, 72